PREVENTION'S BEST
America's #1 Choice for Healthy Living

SYMPTOMS AND SOLUTIONS FOR WOMEN

By the Editors of *Prevention* Health Books

RODALE

ST. MARTIN'S
PAPERBACKS

The information in this book is excerpted from *Women's Edge Health Enhancement Guide: Get Well, Stay Well* (Rodale, 2000), *The Doctors Book of Home Remedies for Seniors* (Rodale, 1999), *Nature's Medicines* (Rodale, 1999), *Symptoms: Their Causes and Cures* (Rodale, 1994), *New Choices in Natural Healing* (Rodale, 1995), *Prevention's Healing with Vitamins* (Rodale, 1996), and *Men's Health Life Improvement Guide: Symptom Solver* (Rodale, 1997).

Prevention's Best is a trademark and *Prevention* Health Books is a registered trademark of Rodale Inc.

SYMPTOMS AND SOLUTIONS FOR WOMEN

Cover Designer: Anne Twomey
Book Designer: Keith Biery

ISBN 0–312–98185-6   paperback

Printed in the United States of America

Rodale/St. Martin's Paperbacks edition published January, 2002

St. Martin's Paperbacks are published by St. Martin's Press, 175 Fifth Avenue, New York, NY 10010.

10 9 8 7 6 5 4 3 2

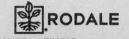

RODALE

WE INSPIRE AND ENABLE PEOPLE TO IMPROVE
THEIR LIVES AND THE WORLD AROUND THEM

Contents

Introduction

When your body wants to send you a message that something is wrong, it sends you a symptom. Symptoms are often painful and usually unpleasant. Do you want to get that message from your body? You bet you do!

Decoding that symptom—figuring out what your body is trying to tell you—is *vital*. Finding out what's causing the symptom often helps you correct something your body's doing wrong. If you're not eating right or getting enough exercise, if you're being exposed to something that's not good for you, your body will let you know by sending you a symptom or two.

Sometimes decoding the symptom/message from your body is easy. In plain English, your "headache" message might read something like: "About that nightcap you had last night: If you *have* to consume alcohol before going to bed—and I would prefer that you didn't—would you kindly have something other than red wine?" Sometimes getting the message is *not* so simple.

That's where this book comes in. It will help you figure out what your symptom is trying to tell you, then help you find out all the possible things you can do about it.

We've made this book easy for you to use. The symptoms are listed in alphabetical order—from A to Z—and we've used popular terms instead of medical jargon. That way you won't have to know that doctors call water retention edema. Just look up "water retention." We realize that people in different parts of the country sometimes have different names for things, so if you don't find what you want at the first try, give a peek at the index at the back of the book.

May your body's symptoms/messages be few and may you "read" them well and use those symptoms to find your way to good health.

PART ONE

Body Talk

Listen to Your Body

Somewhere deep within the recesses of your body is a neglected, ignored voice. It's the voice of a doctor. And it talks to you all the time, diagnosing ailments, recommending treatments, and sometimes making referrals.

"We have to learn to listen to that internal doctor," says Bruce K. Lowell, M.D., an internist and geriatrician in Queens, New York and author of *Body Signals: When to Relax, When to Be Concerned, and When to Go to the Doctor Immediately.*

Your internal doctor uses the language of symptoms to talk with you when something's wrong. A runny nose. An achy elbow. A jackhammer headache. At times, the message is pretty clear, like the burn you feel on your skin after staying out in the sun too long. That's your inner voice's way of telling you to stay in the shade for a while. But other times, the transmission from your body may be scrambled. Dizziness, for example, can be somewhat cryptic. It could mean you're having a stroke. Or it could mean you didn't eat enough for lunch.

Think of symptoms as clues to a mystery and yourself as the bumbling Detective Columbo trying to put together the puzzle pieces before the bad guy strikes again. You can learn to better read the messages your body sends by following these steps.

Educate yourself. You're already ahead of the game on this one because you're reading this book. The more you learn about health, the better you'll understand your body, says Richard Honaker, M.D., of Carrollton, Texas, where he is president of Family Medicine Associates of Texas.

Pay attention. You could be a med school grad, able to identify what every textbook symptom means. But if you

Top 10 Killers of Women

Young Women (Ages 25 to 44)

1. Cancer
2. Accidents
3. Heart disease
4. AIDS
5. Suicide
6. Homicide
7. Stroke
8. Chronic liver disease and cirrhosis
9. Diabetes
10. Pneumonia and influenza

Middle-Aged Women (Ages 45 to 64)

1. Cancer
2. Heart disease
3. Stroke
4. Chronic obstructive pulmonary disease

don't listen to your own body, all that knowledge won't do you a bit of good. The more you stop and listen to your internal doctor, the more you'll realize that you know exactly what's wrong with your body and how to fix it, Dr. Lowell says.

When in doubt, trust the voice. There may be times when your rational side is saying, "It's just a sore throat." But your internal voice is saying, "I don't have a good feeling about this." This will happen more and more often as you age, primarily because the same symptom you had at age 24 does not mean the same thing when you're 54. For instance, stomach pain can have myriad causes. When

  5. Diabetes
  6. Accidents
  7. Chronic liver disease and cirrhosis
  8. Pneumonia and influenza
  9. Suicide
  10. Blood infection

Senior Women (Ages 65 and Up)

  1. Heart disease
  2. Cancer
  3. Stroke
  4. Chronic obstructive pulmonary disease
  5. Pneumonia and influenza
  6. Diabetes
  7. Accidents
  8. Alzheimer's disease
  9. Kidney disease
  10. Blood infection

you're 22, it probably means you have a virus. But at 50, it could mean cancer, says Dr. Lowell.

Take inventory. The best time to do this is when taking a shower. Reflect. Check yourself out. How do you feel? How do you look? "In order to be observant, people need to be intentional about it," says Robert Abel Jr., M.D., clinical professor of ophthalmology at Thomas Jefferson University in Philadelphia, where he is one of the founders of the Alternative Medicine Program and part of a group examining the future of health care.

"You can take the same road to work every day. And one day out of a hundred you stop at a traffic light and notice that there's a place you have never seen before," Dr. Abel says. It's the same way with your body. If you drive it around in an autopilot daze, you're almost certain to miss an important road sign.

Become a body reporter. Even Jimmy Olsen, cub reporter, knows to ask the five Ws and one H: who, what, when, where, why, and how. You can do the same thing with your body, says Dr. Lowell. Ask yourself questions about symptoms. The "who" is obvious. But the other questions certainly apply when a symptom occurs. How long have I had it? When does it happen? What provokes it? Where is it? The questions will do more than just bring you in better touch with your body; they'll also help you describe your symptoms if the pain entails seeing a doctor. "Patients don't have to be physicians. But nothing is worse than when a patient comes in and says, 'Gee, I feel lousy all over.' It means nothing," says Dr. Lowell.

Why We Get Sick

The key to staying healthy is to keep all the aspects of your *selfs*—the physical, emotional, and spiritual—in balance. When you do, you feel and function at your best. You're happy, creative, and productive. You have lots of energy, enjoy strong relationships, and are more able to handle the stressors in your life.

"Some people call it the zone," says Elaine Ferguson, M.D., a holistic physician practicing in Chicago and author of *Healing, Health, and Transformation*. "It's when you've reached the state where you're in harmony."

Illness, on the other hand, is a state of disharmony. You're functioning below your peak because some area of your health is out of balance, says Dr. Ferguson. Perhaps you have a serious illness such as cancer or a chronic disorder such as arthritis, or maybe you simply don't feel your best because of nagging headaches or fatigue.

"I see wellness and sickness as a continuum more than as distinct states," says Marcey Shapiro, M.D., a holistic physician practicing in Albany, California, who specializes in herbal medicine. At one end of the spectrum is optimal

Don't Do That!

When it comes to bad habits, these top the health-endangering list.

Lighting up. Smoking causes emphysema, skin wrinkling, and bone loss in addition to heart disease, lung cancer, and stroke. About 23 percent of women smoke.

Basking in the sun. About 80 percent of skin cancers are caused by sun exposure. Sunbathing also promotes wrinkling and dry skin.

Hitting the sauce too hard. Overconsumption of alcohol has been linked to an increased risk of breast cancer and possibly certain types of stroke, says I-Min Lee, M.D., assistant professor of epidemiology at Harvard School of Public Health. Small amounts are okay since alcohol lowers the risk of heart disease, she says. For optimum

health, and at the other is serious illness. "Very few of us are at the extremes of having ideal health or being terribly ill," she says. "Most of us are somewhere in between."

Heeding the Signs

The symptoms we all get from time to time—stomachaches, insomnia, muscle tension—are warning signs that we're moving away from optimal health. We may not even be sick with a diagnosable illness, but our bodies are trying to tell us that something is out of balance, Dr. Ferguson says.

"We all have this intelligence within our bodies that speaks to us. The message could be a pain or a thought, but our bodies always tell us when something's wrong," Dr. Shapiro says.

health, limit yourself to three to four drinks a week and no more than one drink in a day.

Being a couch potato. A sedentary lifestyle puts you at risk for problems like heart disease, osteoporosis, obesity, and depression, says Lila A. Wallis, M.D., clinical professor of medicine at Weill Medical College of Cornell University. Any motion is better than none. For best results, Dr. Wallis suggests that you regularly engage in a repetitive activity that increases your breathing and heart rate.

Having bad eating habits. A diet high in saturated fat, sugar, and meat and low in vegetables and whole foods is likely to take a negative toll on your body, possibly leading to heart disease, cancer, and chronic gastrointestinal problems.

It's your job to recognize these signs and pay attention to them. Heeding your body's signals will help you get back on the path to optimal health, but first you need to know what signals to watch out for. Here are the common physical, emotional, and mental symptoms that experts say can point to an imbalance in your health.

Muscle tension. Your muscles, especially in your neck, shoulder blades, and back, are full of tight knots.

Fatigue. Your energy level is so low that you just barely get through the day and then crash when you get home from work.

Loss of appetite. You don't feel hungry at mealtimes, and nothing seems appetizing to you.

Weight gain or weight loss. You've dropped or put on several pounds but haven't changed your eating or exercising habits.

Aches and pains. You have frequent, unexplained pain, such as headaches, stomachaches, or heartburn.

Difficulty sleeping. Several nights in a row, you have trouble falling or staying asleep.

Hair loss. You notice more hair than usual in your brush or around the shower drain.

Dizziness or faintness. You feel weak and light-headed, especially when standing up. You may even have fainting spells.

Shortness of breath. You get winded when you walk to your car or up a flight of stairs.

Diarrhea or constipation. Your bowel movements are looser, harder, more frequent, or less frequent than normal.

Anxiety. You feel tense and irritable and can't seem to escape your worries.

Disorganized thoughts. You have difficulty concentrating. You may lose things or forget appointments.

Depression. You are down in the dumps and feel hopeless.

Mood swings. Instead of being your typical pleasant self, you're moody and cranky much of the time.

"These are the signs that happen along the way when we move from optimal health toward illness," says Dr. Shapiro. "Usually, things start out as small whispers that get louder and louder if people don't attend to them."

The problem is that it's easy to blame these symptoms on getting older or on the stresses of everyday life, so we end up dismissing them as quickly as they appear.

"We're so externally focused in terms of how we're taught to think and live that we don't pay attention to our bodies or our inner voices," Dr. Ferguson says. And the more we ignore our bodies, the further away we move from optimal health.

Women's Edge

Some women call it their intuition. Others say it's their sixth sense. Whatever you call it, women are more in touch with their bodies—and that gives them an edge over men when it comes to their health. "Men are taught from childhood to ignore pain rather than to stop and take care of it," says Royda Crose, Ph.D., associate director and associate professor of the Fisher Institute for Wellness and Gerontology at Ball State University in Muncie, Indiana, and author of *Why Women Live Longer Than Men.* Male professional athletes, for example, are notorious for playing while injured.

Women, on the other hand, are good at listening to their bodies. They're better listeners, in part, because the female body requires them to pay attention to its changes. "Our reproductive systems keep us tuned in to our bodies," Dr. Crose says. Because we menstruate, we learn at a young age that our bodies go through constant changes and that we feel physically and emotionally different throughout our cycles. Our periods are just the beginning. Our bodies make sure that we pay attention to them in many other ways as well.

When we get pregnant, for example, our bodies go through constant change for 9 months. During that time, we experience a part of being women that teaches us to be especially in tune with our physical well-being, Dr. Crose points out.

Even when we're not pregnant, most of us have annual gynecological exams and, after 40, mammograms. Eventually, of course, we also experience all the physical changes of menopause, such as hot flashes, mood swings, and the end of our monthly periods. "It's yet another time when our bodies go through changes and we become sensitive to everything that's going on inside of us," Dr. Crose says.

Medicine That Comes in Pink and Blue

Scientists in gender-based biology are discovering that men and women are different at the most basic level, the cellular level. "Women are not just small men," says Sherry Marts, Ph.D., scientific director of the Society for Women's Health Research, based in Washington, D.C.

Researchers studying various drugs began noticing that some work better in women, while others are more effective in men. Take ibuprofen, for example. When it comes to bringing down fevers and inflammation, ibuprofen works about the same in men and women. But it relieves pain much more effectively in men.

The differences don't end there. Diseases affect men and women in different ways as well. "Men tend to get diseases that are more urgent and tend to be more lethal. Women's diseases often start at a slower pace and cause disability long before death," explains Florence Haseltine,

Call a Time-Out

Because all of these physical changes and trips to the doctor make us more aware of what's going on within our bodies, we're in a better position to recognize symptoms of illness when they crop up. But recognizing them isn't enough. We need to act. "When we notice signs that we're not feeling our best, we need to stop and take stock of our lives," Dr. Ferguson says. "I tell my patients to get very quiet and still and to listen and let their bodies tell them what they need to do."

We also need to question ourselves and our habits and examine the things that we've been doing, adds Heather Morgan, M.D., a holistic physician practicing in Centerville, Ohio.

M.D., Ph.D., originator of the term *gender-based biology* and cofounder and former president of the Society for Women's Health Research.

By finding out why autoimmune diseases such as multiple sclerosis are much more common in women and why women develop heart disease decades later than men, we'll learn more about these diseases and develop better treatments for both women and men, Dr. Haseltine says. As a result, someday doctors will treat the same disease differently, depending on the patient's sex, predicts Dr. Marts.

"It will translate itself almost immediately in the cardiac field," Dr. Haseltine says. "But I think the most exciting area of research is the study of structural differences in the brain and how brain disorders such as stroke are treated."

Any number of events can knock us off-kilter. Maybe we have picked up a virus, are grieving the loss of a loved one, or are questioning our spiritual beliefs, Dr. Ferguson says. Perhaps we are under a lot of stress, aren't getting enough sleep, or are routinely passing up nutritious food for high-fat fare. "Everything from our relationships and emotions to what we eat, breathe, and touch affects our health," she says. Our hormones, our expectations, and, of course, our genes all play a role.

Beyond Having Babies

Being female has a great deal of influence over our health. "We're starting to see that there are definitely a lot of physiological differences between men and women," says Sherry Marts, Ph.D., scientific director of the Society for Women's Health Research, based in Washington, D.C. Because our bodies are different than men's, various illnesses and treatments affect us differently as well, she says.

For example, women appear to be more susceptible than men to certain chemical substances, such as alcohol and the carcinogens in cigarettes. Research shows that women develop cirrhosis of the liver after a shorter period of heavy drinking than men do. Women also have a 20 to 70 percent higher risk of developing lung cancer than men at every level of exposure to cigarette smoke. About 75 percent of all people with autoimmune diseases, such as multiple sclerosis and lupus, are female.

When we do get sick, women experience symptoms that are different from men's for the same conditions. A man suffering a heart attack, for example, is likely to have gripping chest pain, while a woman is more likely to have subtle symptoms such as abdominal pain, nausea, and extreme fatigue.

Beyond symptoms, diseases may actually progress differently in men and women. Women with multiple sclerosis, for example, tend to experience periods of remission followed by relapses, while men with the disease tend to have continuously progressive symptoms.

There are even differences between men and women where treatment is concerned. Ibuprofen, for example, is less effective at providing pain relief for women. Women also wake up from anesthesia an average of 4 minutes faster than men.

It all comes down to something most of us intuitively know: To prevent and heal illness, we not only need to keep ourselves in balance but also have to establish health habits that address our special needs.

The Habits of Highly Healthy Women

Although men clearly have physical advantages over women in strength, height, and muscle tone, when it comes to longevity, there's no contest. These days, women outlive men by an average of 5 years—life expectancies are 79 years for women and 74 years for men.

A woman's predisposition to live longer does not, however, mean that she can sit back and enjoy better health with no effort. To gain from the biological advantages, women have to work at taking good care of themselves. Here's a top 10 list of health habits to strive for.

1. Move Your Body

Exercise improves cardiovascular health, which helps prevent heart disease, high blood pressure, and diabetes, explains Sherry Marts, Ph.D., scientific director of the Society for Women's Health Research, based in Washington, D.C. It also helps you look better, have more energy, and be less likely to get depressed. To get the most mileage for your sweat, exercise both aerobically and with weights. "There is also some data showing that weight-bearing exercise prevents osteoporosis, particularly when it's done in your twenties and thirties," she says.

Get your heart pumping. "Walk, and walk faster," says Trudy L. Bush, Ph.D., professor of epidemiology and preventive medicine at the University of Maryland School of Medicine at Baltimore. "All you need is a pair of athletic shoes." For both your heart and your waistline, the American College of Sports Medicine recommends that you exercise aerobically at a moderate pace for 20 to 60 minutes a day 3 to 5 days a week.

Pump yourself up. "Resistance training, such as lifting weights, increases and maintains muscle and bone, which improves body composition and appearance and increases your metabolism," says Jennifer Layne, a certified strength and conditioning specialist and exercise physiologist at the Jean Mayer USDA Human Nutrition Research Center on Aging at Tufts University in Boston. And resistance training builds your strength. The American College of Sports Medicine recommends doing a routine, 2 or 3 days a week, consisting of 8 to 10 exercises that work the major muscle groups. Strive for 8 to 12 repetitions of each exercise.

2. Eat a Healthy, Diverse Diet

A nutritious, varied diet helps lessen your risk of heart disease and certain cancers, such as colon cancer. "Eat lots of fiber, fruits, and vegetables, and a reasonable amount of fat," advises I-Min Lee, M.D., assistant professor of epidemiology at Harvard School of Public Health and assistant professor of medicine at Harvard Medical School. The American Heart Association (AHA) considers no more than 30 percent of daily calories to be a reasonable amount of fat, with less than 10 percent coming from the

Why Women Live Longer Than Men

Here are some possibilities, suggests Royda Crose, Ph.D., associate director and associate professor of the Fisher Institute for Wellness and Gerontology at Ball State University in Muncie, Indiana, and author of *Why Women Live Longer Than Men.*

Testosterone is troublesome. "Testosterone seems to be related to increased activity, impulsiveness, and aggressiveness, which can lead to risky behavior," says Dr. Crose. In their younger years, men are more likely than women to die from accidents, suicide, and homicide. Later in life, testosterone increases bad low-density lipoprotein cholesterol and decreases good high-density lipoproteins, putting men at a greater risk for heart disease.

Estrogen protects. "Medical scientists believe that premenopausal women enjoy a buffering effect from illness, because of estrogen," says Dr. Crose. Estrogen may protect women against heart disease, osteoporosis, and possibly brain disorders like Alzheimer's disease.

Illness gets crossed out. "Scientists believe that females have an advantage in having two X chromosomes, because the second X chromosome provides a backup if something goes wrong with a gene on the first one," says Dr. Crose.

Pears are healthier than apples. Women typically gain weight in their lower bodies—their hips, buttocks, and legs—giving them more of a pear shape, while men are more apple-shaped. "The apple-shaped pattern of obesity is believed to be a strong predictor of increased high blood pressure, diabetes, heart disease, and stroke," says Dr. Crose.

saturated fats contained in animal products. "It's also important to watch your total calorie intake," she says.

Get your fruits and veggies. The AHA recommends that you eat five or more servings of vegetables, fruits, or fruit juices a day. Fruits and vegetables pack lots of vitamins, minerals, and fiber without adding many calories. Ann Gentry, chef and owner of the organic, vegetarian Real Food Daily Restaurant in Los Angeles, recommends that you boost their appeal by buying them fresh and by putting more thought into the way you serve them. "Think color and texture," she says. Put three to five different-colored vegetables on a plate; vary the size and cut. Enhance your diet with unusual items like kale, winter squash, and mangoes.

Control your appetite for critters. The AHA recommends that you keep your daily intake of poultry, fish, or lean meat to no more than 6 ounces. If greasy ribs are your only passion at mealtimes, try using different meats, such as lean cuts of wild game, buffalo, or ostrich, and add flavor with some spices.

Get great flavor from basic spices. "Use basil, oregano, thyme, rosemary, and cilantro," Gentry suggests. She also suggests cooking with miso, which is a soybean paste. "Whether you're making soups, pastes, sauces, or spreads, miso can really go a long way."

3. Bone Up on Calcium

Osteoporosis (brittle bones) affects 20 million American women, and one of the best ways to prevent the disease is with calcium. Here's how to boost your intake.

Dine on some dairy. "Eat yogurt and other calcium-rich foods," says Dr. Bush. The National Institutes of Health suggests that you get 1,000 to 1,500 milligrams of calcium daily. Try to choose nonfat or low-fat dairy products such as fat-free milk or low-fat cheese.

Supplement it. "Most Americans don't get enough calcium," says Dr. Lee. To up your intake, turn to supplements. But keep your total daily intake from diet and supplements below 2,500 milligrams, says Lila A. Wallis, M.D., clinical professor of medicine at Weill Medical College of Cornell University in New York City and co-author of *The Whole Woman*. Higher doses must be taken under medical supervision.

4. Get Enough Sleep

"Sleep deprivation may reduce your body's defenses and increase your risk of disease," says Dr. Lee. It's believed that when you fall asleep, infection-fighting blood cells move from your bloodstream into your tissues, attacking viruses and bacteria as you snooze.

Sleep deprivation can also affect your emotional well-being. You may be more testy, and your attention span may suffer, says Rosalind Cartwright, Ph.D., director of the Sleep Disorder Service and Research Center at Rush–Presbyterian–St. Luke's Medical Center in Chicago. Here are suggestions to help you improve your sleep patterns.

Replace lost hormones if you are postmenopausal. "Since the hormones we lose at menopause are implicated in the breathing disorders of sleep, supplementation is a good idea," says Dr. Cartwright. "Hormone supplements also reduce sleep disturbances caused by hot flashes."

Stick to a regular schedule. "If you don't sleep long enough one night, don't go to bed earlier the next night," says Dr. Cartwright. Going to sleep and getting up at the same time every day will help establish a regular sleep/wake cycle.

Behave yourself before bedtime. Your activities immediately before you hit the sack can interfere with your sleep. "Avoid heavy meals or booze before bedtime," says Dr. Cartwright. Heavy meals could cause heartburn, and alcohol,

Eat These for Better Health

Consuming more organic, natural products can help you maintain your health, says Jennifer Brett, N.D., a naturopathic physician in Stratford, Connecticut. Here are some health-building foods to add to your shopping list.

- *Amaranth.* It is a near-complete protein, loaded with calcium and other vital nutrients. Available as a seed, flour, or puffed.
- *Arrowroot.* Use instead of cornstarch (which may cause constipation, diarrhea, and vitamin loss) as a thickening agent in recipes.
- *Cayenne.* A good seasoning, this red pepper helps break up mucus and cholesterol. It also may improve circulation. An excellent substitute for black pepper, it is available in mild, medium, and hot varieties.
- *Eggs.* Purchase free-range or organic for better taste and no hormones.

although it makes you drowsy, will wake you up about 3 hours later. And although walking has been shown to promote good sleep, don't work out less than 4 hours before hitting the sack, because exercise's stimulating effects may keep you up.

If you must nap, keep it short. "If you need to extend your waking hours, a 15- to 20-minute nap midday will help," says Dr. Cartwright. "Longer naps make you wake up with a 'sleep hangover' and may interfere with your sleep that night."

5. Stop Stressing

"Stress results from the perception that you are ill-equipped to meet the demands on your mind and body," says Mar-

- *Foods for liver health.* Beets, carrots, artichokes, lemons, parsnips, dandelion greens, and watercress all help keep your liver healthy.
- *Millet.* This tasty gluten-free whole grain is very nutritious and easy to digest.
- *Nutritional yeast.* Yeasts, such as brewer's, are stocked with nutrients, including B vitamins. Sprinkle on popcorn, bread, and cereal.
- *Spelt.* This member of the wheat family can often be tolerated by people with gluten or wheat allergies and by people with celiac disease. It contains more protein and fiber than wheat.
- *Stevia.* Also known as honey leaf, it's an herbal sweetener without the side effects of artificial sweeteners. Just one to three drops is plenty to sweeten a cup of tea.

garet Caudill, M.D., Ph.D., codirector of the department of pain medicine at Dartmouth-Hitchcock Medical Center in Manchester, New Hampshire. Stress can also result from an overload of positive activities, such as when planning a wedding. "Unchecked stress can cause decreased sleep, muscle tension, heart palpitations, shortness of breath, and irritable bowel symptoms," she says. Long-term stress may lead to the development of chronic health problems such as high blood pressure and decreased immune function. To help de-stress yourself, consider this advice.

Listen up. "It's important to identify your stress symptoms," says Dr. Caudill. Most of us know how we react to stress—a tense neck, stomach pain, lack of sleep, irritability. The key is to home in on the symptoms early so you can quickly take steps to deal with the stressful situation that's causing them.

Do something for yourself. Don't nurture everyone else at the expense of your own needs. Make a commitment to yourself, says Dr. Caudill. "Do something on a regular basis to relieve tension." It doesn't take much—get some exercise or just take a few deep breaths.

Meditate. "Repeatedly focusing on a word, phrase, breath, or motion can cause the relaxation response during and after meditation, which can reduce stress-related changes in your body," says Dr. Caudill. Meditate once a day for 10 to 20 minutes to rejuvenate both your body and your mind.

6. Pay Your Doctor a Visit

Yearly exams can prevent a number of conditions, including breast and cervical cancers and osteoporosis, says Dr. Wallis. Have your body screened with these tests.

Get a mammogram. "The mortality rate from breast cancer is decreasing, which is probably related to the detection of early lesions by mammogram," says Paula Szypko, M.D., a pathologist at North State Pathology Associates in High Point, North Carolina, and spokesperson for the College of American Pathologists. Premalignant and early noninvasive tumors can be detected by a mammogram before they can be felt. Dr. Szypko suggests going for an annual mammogram every year after age 40. "In addition, do monthly self-examinations and have an annual examination by your health-care practitioner," she says.

Prevent cancer with a Pap test. "The death rate from uterine cervical cancers has dropped significantly since the Pap test became available almost 50 years ago," says Dr. Szypko. The preventive effects of the test are tremendous. Eighty percent of women who die of cervical cancer have not had a Pap test in 5 years. She recommends that you have an annual Pap test starting at age 18. "A lot of women believe that they don't need to have Pap tests if they're beyond their childbearing years, but 60 percent of cervical cancers occur in women over age 55," she says.

Give the rest of your body a once-over. In addition to a Pap test and mammogram, you should have an annual flu shot and cholesterol and blood pressure checks, says Dr. Bush. Women over 45 should have a dual-energy x-ray absorptiometry (DEXA) bone scan to check for osteoporosis. If you're over 50, you should also undergo a screening for rectal and colon cancers every 5 to 10 years.

7. Buckle Up

There's really no excuse for not spending the 3 to 7 seconds it takes to fasten your seat belt. If you still refuse to buckle up when you're driving alone, at least buckle up in front of your children. If you don't, you send a message that it's okay to go without a seat belt.

And remember that *all* passengers should buckle up. The American College of Emergency Physicians states that in a 55-mile-per-hour crash, an unrestrained backseat passenger could fly forward at a force strong enough to seriously injure or even kill a person in the front.

Finally, make sure that you're buckled properly. According to the AAA, a seat belt worn incorrectly could do more harm than good. The belt should be over your hips and pelvis, in front of your chest, and over your shoulder. A belt worn behind your body could cause your head to hit the dashboard, and a belt worn under your arm could break your ribs and lead to serious internal injuries.

8. Renew Your Relationships

"People who are emotionally connected to other people do better in terms of disease risk than people who are not connected," says Dr. Lee. The effects of isolation are even worse for people with chronic illness. People with coronary artery disease who have spouses or confidantes, for example, are 30 percent more likely to survive than patients who are isolated. Here are a few ways you can stay connected.

Build a support network. "People with good social health have relationships that are interdependent and complementary, where each person helps the other," says Royda Crose, Ph.D., associate director and associate professor of the Fisher Institute for Wellness and Gerontology at Ball State University in Muncie, Indiana, and author of *Why Women Live Longer Than Men.* "Such interdependent relationships provide a safety net that's important for survival throughout life but is especially crucial in old age."

Keep your love alive. To remain zestful, love relationships need a constant supply of fresh energy. Be spontaneous with your partner, whether you make a last-minute decision to walk in the park or to fly to the Bahamas. And remember to laugh—it boosts the joyful spirit that connected you in the first place, says Dr. Crose.

Explore your spirituality. Religious activities can give meaning to your life and provide personal satisfaction outside your family. "Spiritual and religious connections provide motivation and hope—outlooks that promote longevity," says Dr. Crose.

9. Laugh Out Loud

Laughter is the physiological response to humor. Research suggests that laughter produces benefits like increased antibodies, decreased stress hormones, and a higher pain threshold. "Laughter is also good for your emotional health," says Dr. Bush.

According to a study done at Loma Linda University in California, when heart attack patients added a 30-minute humorous video to their cardiac rehabilitation, they had lower blood pressure, fewer stress hormones, and lower medication requirements.

10. Have a Hobby

Doing an activity for your own sake provides a source of enjoyment that can reduce stress and improve well-being, says Dr. Bush. To incorporate a new activity into your life, try the following.

Look back to your youth. Renew a hobby you had earlier, whether it's painting, playing cards, or even mall walking; if you enjoyed it before, take it up again.

Dig in the dirt. Garden work has been shown to spark creativity and optimism, and physically, it burns calories and can lower blood pressure.

Volunteer. "I think that volunteering, the idea of altruism, is important," says Dr. Caudill. "It's been demonstrated that people who make connections with people and do things for others are healthier."

By volunteering, you can enhance your own life as you learn new skills and form new relationships, says Dr. Crose.

Lines of Defense

Our doctors aren't spending much time with us. In fact, a typical primary-care physician spends less than 13 minutes with each patient every 6 months.

That doesn't leave much time for the kind of basic preventive medicine that can help to keep us healthy. In a 1998 survey conducted by the Commonwealth Fund, only 55 percent of women reported that their blood cholesterol had been tested in the previous year. Nearly 40 percent said that they had not had physical exams or Pap tests. One in three had not undergone clinical breast exams. And one in six had not received any preventive care during that time.

But time is not the only problem. "Physicians traditionally are not taught how to be good prevention counselors," says Linda Hyder Ferry, M.D., associate professor of preventive medicine and family medicine at Loma Linda University School of Medicine in California. So, like it or not, the burden of responsibility for preventive care rests primarily on our own shoulders.

"Women must become consumer advocates for themselves. They need to read everything they can about preventive care because most physicians aren't likely to provide the best prevention strategies," Dr. Ferry says.

Eat Good Food to Sidetrack Ailments

The USDA Food Guide Pyramid is an excellent foundation for helping people prevent many illnesses, says Jennifer Brett, N.D., a naturopathic physician in Stratford, Connecticut. The pyramid says that women should eat 6 to 11 servings daily of bread, cereal, rice, and pasta; 2 to 4 servings of fruits, such as apples, strawberries, and bananas; 3 to 5 servings of vegetables, such as broccoli, tomatoes, and lettuce; 2 to 3 servings of milk, yogurt, cheese, and other dairy products; and 2 to 3 servings of meat, poultry, fish, dried beans, eggs, or nuts. Fats should be used sparingly. But the pyramid is just one of many tools that women should use to maintain their health.

"Your entire health derives from what you do every day. All the pills in the world aren't going to make up for a bad foundation," Dr. Brett says. "Of course, there are specific needs for individuals. A woman with recurring yeast infections, for instance, might help herself prevent those infections if she eats foods that contain less sugar, starch, and other refined carbohydrates."

Although every woman's dietary needs differ slightly, here are a few general guidelines that can help keep you in peak nutritional condition.

Peel me a grape. Bite into the fresh fruits and vegetables that you enjoy, experiment with new ones, and eat a variety of all of them, Dr. Brett urges. The phytochemicals (plant chemicals) they contain may help ward off such catastrophic diseases as cancer, heart disease, and stroke. Researchers suspect that various mixtures of compounds neutralize free radicals, those unstable molecules that damage or destroy healthy cells. Since phytochemicals work as groups, you need a lot of them to make a difference. No single fruit or vegetable contains all you need. The greater the variety of produce you consume, the better off you will be.

Snap up beans. Navy, pinto, lima, and other dried beans are virtually fat-free and are tremendous sources of protein that can slash or even eliminate the need for fat-laden meats in chili, stews, and salads.

To cut down on gas, soak your beans overnight in a bowl of water, then use fresh water for cooking them.

Your Tree of Knowledge

Research your family history of ailments by talking to your parents, grandparents, aunts, uncles, and siblings. If a blood relative has a disease or condition, you need not panic, but you should be aware that you are at an increased risk.

Serious but potentially preventable conditions are the ones you should pay the most attention to, including cancer, high blood pressure, diabetes, alcoholism, heart disease, and depression.

Organize your findings into a simple family tree chart so you can view the medical histories of several relatives all at once. Assign a letter to each medical condition or disease that occurs in your family and place that letter under each affected relative. Develop a key to note which conditions the letters represent. Also note the age of death if the relative is deceased.

When your medical family tree is as complete as you can make it, review it with your physician to get a clearer understanding of your risks.

Over-the-counter products such as Beano also can help prevent gas by breaking down sugars in your digestive system.

Don't let meat hog your plate. Limit yourself to no more than 6 ounces of cooked meat a day. Use a small portion (2 to 3 ounces after cooking) to complement, not dominate, each meal. Or think of it this way: For every bite of meat, take four bites of fruits, vegetables, beans, and grains.

Sneak in soy. Soy contains isoflavones: substances that block the formation of blood vessels around new tumors, stop cancer cells from multiplying, and prevent the absorption of tumor-promoting estrogen. So instead of beef, chicken, and other meats, use soy products like tofu as a main course in your meals.

Wear a milk mustache. Milk is fortified with vitamin D, which your body needs to absorb calcium. Calcium helps prevent osteoporosis, a degenerative bone disease. Drinking 2½ to 3 glasses of fat-free milk a day can help you reach a goal of 1,000 milligrams through your diet. Other good sources of calcium include yogurt, Cheddar cheese, sardines (with bones), tofu, and calcium-fortified orange juice.

Take your breath away. Eating half an onion or a clove of garlic a day helps regulate bacteria and other organisms in both your intestines and reproductive tract. Both onion and garlic also contain a great number of antioxidant compounds that fight cancer and heart disease.

Heave hydrogenated foods. Commercial baked goods and margarine are often loaded with hydrogenated or partially hydrogenated oils. This means that hydrogen has been added to unsaturated fat to make it solidify. This process creates saturated fat and trans fatty acids—a gruesome pairing that raises blood levels of low-density lipoproteins (LDL), the bad cholesterol that clogs arteries.

Be a Health Detective

Resources abound for getting information about your health or a particular illness. Here are books you can find at the library, followed by Web sites you can check there or at home.

- *Mayo Clinic Family Health Book* and *The American Medical Association Family Medical Guide* provide basic health information in easy-to-understand language.
- *Health Care Almanac: Every Person's Guide to the Thoughtful and Practical Sides of Medicine,* by the American Medical Association, is arranged in alphabetical order with addresses of medical associations and a variety of health-related information.
- *The Female Body: An Owner's Manual,* by the editors of *Prevention* Magazine Health Books, covers concerns women have about their health.
- *Our Bodies, Ourselves for the New Century,* by the Boston Women's Health Book Collective staff, provides women with comprehensive coverage of health care.

So if you read the word *hydrogenated* on a food label, put the package back on the grocery shelf.

Reach for a supplement. Getting adequate amounts of all the nutrients that you need to stay healthy can be a challenge, so take a once-a-day multivitamin. It should include 100 percent of the Daily Values for calcium, magnesium, niacin, iron, folic acid, chromium, and vitamins A, C, D, E, and B_{12}. The antioxidant vitamins in these preparations will help prevent heart disease and other tissue damage.

- Healthfinder (www.healthfinder.gov), a government Web site, offers a searchable database with additional links to professional organizations, academic institutions, and libraries.
- The American College of Obstetricians and Gynecologists (www.acog.org) addresses a variety of women's health issues.
- CancerNet (http://cancernet.nci.nih.gov), from the National Cancer Institute, provides current cancer information covering diagnosis, treatment, and cancer physicians and facilities.
- The National Women's Health Information Center (www.4woman.org) is maintained by the U.S. Department of Health and Human Services and has updated health-related news stories, consumer information, and links to medical dictionaries and glossaries.
- The North American Menopause Society (www.menopause.org) discusses scientific studies related to menopause.

Jump-Start Your Exercise Routine

Regular exercise can reduce the risk of heart disease and stroke among women. In addition, women who exercise an hour a day may also reduce their risk of breast cancer by 20 percent, according to findings from the Nurses' Health Study, one of the largest studies ever done on women's health. Other researchers who evaluated data from the Nurses' Health Study found that women who did the most weekly exercise had significantly lower risks of developing type 2 diabetes than women who exercised the least.

Weight-bearing exercise, such as walking, jogging, and running, can also help women maintain bone mass and derail osteoporosis, says Marianne Legato, M.D., founder and director of the Partnership for Women's Health at Columbia University College of Physicians and Surgeons in New York City and author of *What Women Need to Know*.

Simply walking 40 minutes a day, four times a week, can make an enormous difference in your body's ability to defend itself against a multitude of ailments.

Rest Easy

Sleep helps your body rebuild muscle tissue and replenish chemicals in your brain. Taking 200 to 300 milligrams of both calcium and magnesium every evening can help you get more restful sleep, Dr. Brett says.

Valerian, an herbal remedy, can have tranquilizing and sedative properties similar to the prescription drug diazepam (Valium), but without the side effects. Plus, valerian is nonaddictive. Dr. Brett suggests taking two 400-milligram capsules 30 minutes before bedtime. Valerian is also sold as a tea, but Dr. Brett says it can be difficult to drink. Do not use valerian with sleep-enhancing or mood-regulating medications because it may intensify their effects. It may cause heart palpitations and nervousness in sensitive individuals. If it stimulates you that way, discontinue use. Valerian is available at health food stores.

In addition, heed the following advice to sleep better.

Stick to a schedule. Try to go to bed and wake up at approximately the same times each day.

Kick back and unwind. Take a few moments before you turn in to unload the stresses of the day through meditation or deep breathing.

Drink milk or herbal tea. Milk is loaded with L-tryptophan, which helps some people sleep. Drinking

The Warning Signs of Cancer

Caught early, many cancers can be subdued. Here are the signals to look for, according to the American Cancer Society.

- Any change in bowel or bladder habits
- A sore that does not heal
- A lump or thickening in the breast or elsewhere
- Unusual bleeding or discharge
- Chronic indigestion or swallowing problems
- An obvious change in a wart or a mole
- A nagging cough or hoarseness

In most cases, these signs are symptoms of some disease other than cancer. But to be on the safe side, if you notice any of them, notify your doctor immediately. If it does turn out that you have cancer, the sooner you get started on treatment, the better your chances will be for a complete recovery and a long, healthy life.

herb tea before bed is a soothing ritual that can help you relax.

Avoid alcohol and caffeine. Taken up to 8 hours before bed, either will disrupt your natural sleep patterns.

Eat light. A large dinner or late-night snack might keep you tossing and turning as your digestive tract works overtime.

Strangle Stress

Among the most stressed women in the world are full-time working mothers with children under the age of 13, with nearly one in four feeling stress almost every day. More single women than single men around the world feel intense daily stress, and the number of stressed separated or divorced women exceeds that of similar men by a three-to-two margin.

Of course, excessive stress is more than just a nuisance. It can make women more susceptible to infections and hormonal imbalances, Dr. Brett says. Meditation, yoga, and other techniques can go a long way toward reducing the stress that you feel and, in turn, reduce your risk of disease.

Listening to music is the number one stress-buster for more than half of the world's women. Reading, walking, and taking a bath or shower are other popular ways to unwind.

Make an Annual Pilgrimage

Regular physical exams and medical tests can help detect small problems in your body before they get big. The type and number of tests you need each year depend on many factors, including your age and previous medical history. But here are a few critical tests that women older than 40 should undergo, according to Dr. Legato.

- A blood pressure reading by a doctor or nurse at least once a year. High blood pressure (readings consistently above 140/90) is a risk factor for stroke and heart disease.
- A mammogram at least every other year after age 40 to help detect breast cancer.
- A manual breast exam by a knowledgeable physician once a year.
- A complete head-to-toe skin exam by a knowledgeable physician once a year.
- A cholesterol screening once a year. Since heart disease is the number one killer of women, Dr. Legato believes that monitoring total cholesterol, LDL,

high-density lipoproteins (HDL), and triglycerides is
an essential component of preventive care.

- A thyroid-function test every year after age 50. For
this test, your blood sample is analyzed at a laboratory.
- A bone-density screening to help determine your risk
of developing osteoporosis. You only have to have
this test done once.
- A serum estradiol test every 2 years after age 45.
Low blood levels of estradiol (less than 50 pico-
grams/deciliter) may mean that you need hormone-
replacement therapy.
- An electrocardiogram (EKG) every year. More than
one in three heart attacks that occur in women are
silent, without any outward warning signals. An EKG
can help determine if you've had any heart damage
in the previous year.
- A fecal occult blood test every year after age 50. This
test can disclose any hidden blood in your stool that
may be a warning sign of colon cancer and other diseases.
- A digital rectal exam once a year to feel for growths,
abnormalities, and signs of bleeding.

In between these tests, always be sure to do monthly
skin and breast self-examinations at home, Dr. Ferry urges.

Choose Your Team

Many of us spend more time and effort on locating a good hairdresser than on finding a good doctor. But finding the right doctor is something we all need to do—now, when we're well, not when we're on the way to the hospital.

For women, there are special health issues that doctors should be familiar with. Can your doctor, for instance, give female-specific advice about preventing heart disease? Can she answer your questions about hormone-replacement therapy? Does she know enough about alternative medicine—herbs, supplements, and the like—to have an intelligent conversation with you about any alternative treatments you are using? Maybe you have both a regular and an alternative doctor. Wouldn't it be wonderful if the two of them could talk together about your care once in a while? Here's how to make that happen.

Finding Dr. Right

Nowadays, two types of doctors perform the role formerly played by the general practitioner: the family practitioner and the internist. While doctors in both of these specialties receive similar training, there are some significant differences between them.

Family practitioners study general adult medicine as well as pediatrics, gynecology, obstetrics, and in-office surgical procedures. So their training is broad. Internists, on the other hand, receive more in-depth training in the diagnosis and treatment of adult illnesses, such as diabetes and heart disease.

Gynecologists sometimes act as primary-care doctors for women. They can offer some preventive care, monitor your blood pressure and cholesterol, and do screening tests for thyroid function and colon cancer. But gynecology is actually a medical-surgical specialty, and a gynecologist's skills are best used to treat illness of your reproductive organs.

One of the best ways to find a competent doctor is to ask around. If you can, question people who work in the medical field. Emergency room physicians and nurses are often in a good position to judge the abilities of local doctors. If it's a gynecologist you're after, ask midwives and nurse practitioners, says Karla Morales, vice president of communications for People's Medical Society, a nonprofit organization devoted to consumer health issues, in Allentown, Pennsylvania.

Doctor-referral services can also be somewhat helpful, but you need to be aware of their limitations. Listed in the yellow pages, these services are usually run either by a local hospital, which lists only doctors employed there, or by a county medical society, which is a paid-membership organization.

At the least-sophisticated level, these services simply give callers the names of doctors from a rotating list of members. The better services, on the other hand, list basic information concerning board certification and specialties of their doctors. And most of them weed out doctors who have been the subject of numerous complaints. "But these services do not give true comparisons or negative information about doctors," says Morales. For that information, contact the American Board of Medical Specialties at 1007 Church Street, Suite 404, Evanston, IL 60201.

A Male or Female Doctor?

It's true that female doctors are more likely than male doctors to offer advice on preventing illness. They also tend to be better listeners and are less likely to interrupt their patients. But, on average, they rate only slightly better—10 percent—at these skills than male doctors. In fact, differences among female doctors are often greater than the average difference between male and female doctors.

So making female gender your number one priority when you're doctor shopping isn't necessarily going to find you the best doctor in your area. It's probably better to look for a doctor, male or female, who encourages you to ask questions, listens to you, explains things clearly, and treats you with respect.

However, when it comes to intimate personal examinations, women and men tend to be more comfortable and more frank with someone of their own gender and ethnicity. A woman who is uncomfortable with a pelvic or breast examination usually prefers seeing a female gynecologist for her care. Maybe that's one reason that female doctors now make up the majority of gynecologists.

Expert consulted: Erica Frank, M.D., associate professor in the department of family and preventive medicine at Emory University School of Medicine in Atlanta

Taking the Alternate Route

If you're looking for a doctor practicing alternative medicine, consider a naturopathic doctor (N.D.). An N.D. is trained in all forms of alternative medicine, including nutrition and herbal remedies. Look for one who is a member of the American Association of Naturopathic Physicians (AANP). These doctors have all graduated from one of the four U.S. or Canadian colleges recognized by the Council on Naturopathic Medical Education.

Check the AANP's Web site at www.naturopathic.org. For a small fee, you can receive a national membership list and a brochure describing naturopathic physicians and their services from the AANP, 601 Valley Street, Suite 105, Seattle, WA 98109-4229.

Eleven states license naturopathic doctors, and four states (Connecticut, Montana, Washington, and Alaska) require that health insurance providers cover N.D. care. In other states, anyone can claim to be a naturopathic doctor, so checking credentials and education is important.

What about Dentists?

If you're looking for a dentist, experts again suggest that you ask for help from people you know and trust, including health-care professionals such as your doctor. You can also call to ask faculty members of the nearest dental school, which is often associated with a medical school. About three out of four dentists also belong to the American Dental Association (ADA), which means that they have some interest in continuing education and maintaining a professional practice, says Kimberly Harms, D.D.S., a dentist from Farmington, Minnesota, and consumer advisor for the ADA. The ADA can give you a list of its members in your area. Contact them at ADA, 211 East Chicago Avenue, Chicago, IL 60611. You can also request information via e-mail on their Web site at www.ada.org.

The staff of the dentist's office should allow you to come in to look around or to have a get-acquainted visit with the dentist, where you simply discuss your concerns and get to know each other, Dr. Harms says. A good dentist will have a clean, organized office and friendly staff; will use proper sterilization techniques, including wearing

Mammograms for the Small-Busted

Although smaller-breasted women may be concerned about whether an adequate mammogram can be done on them, they should be assured that the size of their breasts doesn't matter, even if they are A or AA cups. Technicians seldom have to treat small-breasted women differently from women who have larger breasts. The compression is the same. It doesn't hurt any more or less if you have smaller breasts.

But the truly important message here is for small-breasted women to get annual mammograms after age 40 like everyone else. Some women with smaller breasts may think that they are at lower risk for cancer because they have less breast tissue. But that's not true. Breast cancer is no more common among large-breasted women than among smaller-breasted women. No matter how much breast tissue she has, every woman has the same percentage of risk as any other woman in her age group.

Expert consulted: Deborah Capko, M.D., breast surgeon and associate medical director at the Institute for Breast Care at Hackensack University Medical Center in New Jersey a face mask and gloves; will take a comprehensive dental and medical history before working on you; and will openly discuss treatment options and fees, she says. Many dentists these days work with a dental hygienist, who cleans your teeth, so you'll want to meet the dental hygienist as well.

By the way, D.D.S. and D.M.D. degrees are basically the same thing.

Does Your Doctor Have the Right Stuff?

Whether the doctor is traditional or alternative, you need to check her credentials and other more subjective aspects of her practice, says Morales. Call the doctor's office for this information. It's a good way to find out if her staff is consumer-friendly and willing to answer your questions. Here are some questions you should ask.

- Is the doctor accepting new patients?
- Is the doctor board-certified? Board certification means that the doctor has taken extra training and passed the rigorous examination given by a national board of professionals in that specialty field. Board certification is an important way by which doctors judge their colleagues' credentials. Keep in mind that alternative physicians are not likely to be board-certified.
- Does the doctor have get-acquainted visits? How long are they? (Expect 10 to 15 minutes.) How much do they cost?
- At what hospitals does the doctor have privileges to admit, treat, or operate on her patients? Privileges are rights granted to a doctor by a hospital review board, depending on the hospital's need for doctors and on a doctor's qualifications.

Hospitals Can Make You Sick

It's ironic that people sometimes go into the hospital well and come out sick. The reason: Hospitals are full of sick people, and sick people are sometimes contagious. Organisms can be transmitted in the air, by direct human contact, on towels and sheets, via the housekeeping crew, by contact with surgical wounds, and through the use of urinary catheters, drainage tubes, and ventilator tubes. Studies show that most people don't develop a hospital-acquired infection until at least 72 hours after admission, so some infections may not become apparent until after you've been discharged from the hospital.

How can you protect yourself? Ask your doctor about the hospital's track record for infections. (People at the hospital itself may paint too rosy a picture.) Make sure all hospital personnel who come in contact with you wash their hands. Ask them to do so in your room, in your presence.

Nurses who wear fake fingernails are more likely to harbor harmful organisms than those who don't. In one

- Does the doctor accept phone calls from patients? At what hours? Does she have e-mail? The doctor's staff can frequently answer questions over the phone, but you should have access to the doctor herself if you feel that's necessary.
- Does she have any evening or weekend hours?
- How far in advance is the doctor booked for routine appointments? How quickly can you get in for an emergency?
- Does the doctor work in a group? How many doctors are in the group? Are they all board-certified? Who backs up the doctor when she's on vacation?

study, 68 percent of nurses wearing fake nails were carrying harmful bacteria on their hands even after washing, so ask nurses who wear fake nails to put on gloves before treating you.

If you're concerned that a sick roommate has something you could catch, ask your doctor or nurse about your risk. Change your room at once if there is any chance that you could become infected.

If you're undergoing a procedure that requires the removal of hair, refuse to be shaven the night before surgery. A low rate of infection is achieved by using a chemical depilatory or barber clippers to remove hair on the morning of the surgery.

If you have a urinary catheter, a nurse should check it regularly to make sure that it is draining correctly. This may help you avoid a urinary tract infection.

Expert consulted: Karla Morales, vice president of communications for People's Medical Society

- Does she work in conjunction with alternative practitioners or make referrals to them?

When You Should Fire Your Doctor

What if you're seeing a doctor you just don't care for? No doctor is perfect. You may want to discuss your dissatisfactions with her before you start shopping for a new doctor. There may be room for reconciliation.

Still, most experts say that it's time to end the relationship if your doctor puts you down or judges you, fails to exercise good medical judgment, orders the same test several times when once would do, does not perform thorough physical exams, or minimizes serious side effects or risks of a treatment. Likewise, think about going elsewhere if your doctor blocks your attempts at communication, makes you feel so intimidated that you don't speak up, isn't interested in your worries and concerns, ignores psychological and social causes of illness as well as job-related health problems, or is disrespectful or verbally abusive to you or others.

PART TWO

The Symptoms

Afternoon Slump

You rise and shine with the new day, ready to take on the world. You roll through your morning tasks like a ball of fire. And then in the afternoon, you fizzle.

This sudden slump is a normal, healthy, expected function of our circadian rhythms—the built-in biological clocks that regulate our sleep/wake systems, explains biological psychologist David F. Dinges, Ph.D., associate professor in the psychiatry department at the University of Pennsylvania School of Medicine in Philadelphia.

"In the mornings, we are refreshed after a night's sleep, and our energy and alertness are at peak levels," says Dr. Dinges. "There is a dip in the middle of the afternoon when sleepiness reappears—our natural nap zone. Later in the afternoon, our alertness typically rises again."

Individuals differ in the degree to which this slump hits. Generally, the depth of the dip is a function of how sleepy you are and the amount of sleep you get at night. "If you are short on sleep and in an inactive situation, alertness will go down and you'll really feel sleepiness creep in—usually between 1:00 and 3:00 P.M.," says Wilse

B. Webb, Ph.D., professor of psychology at the University of Florida in Gainesville. "If the slump hits you extremely hard, it could just mean that you have an extremely strong nap tendency. But it could also mean that you are chronically depriving yourself of adequate restorative sleep at night."

Your noontime meal can also lead you into an afternoon tailspin. Bonnie J. Spring, Ph.D., professor of psychology at the University of Health Sciences/Chicago Medical School, has shown in studies that a high-carbohydrate/low-protein lunch can produce an afternoon drop in energy and alertness by elevating the brain's levels of serotonin, a substance that makes us sleepy.

Here are some energy boosters you can use to recharge your battery and give the afternoon slump the slip.

Take a walk. A rapid 10-minute walk raises energy faster and to a greater degree than sweets and snacks, according to Robert Thayer, Ph.D., professor of psychology at California State University in Long Beach. "A general body arousal occurs, which activates a number of different systems in the mind and body to produce an uplifting effect for up to 2 hours," he says.

Take a nap. If your situation allows, catch a couple of winks. "A brief nap can be quite invigorating," says Dr. Webb. "A good rule for naps is that they should never be longer than 1 hour and never occur after 4:00 P.M."

Get plenty of sleep the night before. "If you are sleep deprived, you're more likely to be hit hard by the circadian dip," says Dr. Dinges. Getting adequate sleep at night and maintaining regular sleep patterns can lessen its severity.

Rearrange your schedule. Schedule more passive activities like driving, reading, and paperwork for the morning and late afternoon when your alertness is high, suggests Dr. Dinges. "Use the slump period for engaging in busier social activities like talking on the phone, interacting with coworkers, and doing physical tasks," he says.

Don't skip breakfast. "Skipping breakfast creates a big energy gap that you'll feel all day, even if you eat a good lunch," says James A. Corea, Ph.D., a registered physical therapist in Moorestown, New Jersey, and former trainer with the Philadelphia Eagles football team. "Start with a decent-size, low-fat breakfast of cereal, fresh fruit, whole wheat toast, and skim milk. You can't go wrong."

Eat a balanced lunch. The ideal lunch is a balance of proteins and carbohydrates. A good example of a slump-fighting, high-energy lunch would consist of any combination of fish, pasta, rice, baked potato, fruit salad, vegetable, lean meat, or soup, according to Dr. Corea.

Avoid the lunchtime martini. Alcohol is a depressant, and like many other drugs, it can hit you like a ton of bricks.

Avoid sugary snacks. "After a brief energy surge, sugar produces increased tiredness," says Dr. Thayer. Candy bars and junk food may be convenient, but they can actually drag your slump down deeper. Fresh fruit and popcorn make more reliable snacks.

Drink coffee or soda. Caffeine is a powerful stimulant that can get you through this time period, says Philip R. Westbrook, M.D., director of the Sleep Disorders Center at Cedars-Sinai Medical Center in Los Angeles. Be careful not to overdo the coffee in the morning—the lift you get from more than four cups can send you crashing down in the early afternoon, making the dip even worse.

Anal Itching

The causes of anal itching are numerous, and finding a specific reason for it can be elusive, doctors say. More than likely, hemorrhoids, pinworms, fissures (cracks in the skin surrounding the anus), anal warts, or allergic reactions to toilet paper or foods are responsible for your dilemma. Anal itching also can be caused by a fungal infection, which is particularly common among people with diabetes and can be one of the first signs of the disease.

"I would be wary of using over-the-counter creams and ointments to deal with anal itching. They may do more harm than good, and frankly, there are easier ways of dealing with it," says Bruce Orkin, M.D., an assistant professor specializing in colon and rectal surgery at the George Washington University School of Medicine and Health Sciences in Washington, D.C. Here are a few suggestions on how to banish that tormenting itch from your life.

Nix citrus fruits and spicy foods. Doctors aren't sure why, but citrus fruits, such as oranges, grapefruits, and tangerines, and spicy foods, like curry and hot peppers, can cause some people to develop irritating secretions at the anus, says Juan Nogueras, M.D., a colon and rectal surgeon at the Cleveland Clinic-Florida in Fort Lauderdale. Simply eliminating these foods from your diet may solve the problem, he says.

Try a fruit cocktail. Besides adding fiber to the diet, which softens the stool, a number of fruit juices contain substances that may help ease hemorrhoids, says Cherie Calbom, M.S., a certified nutritionist in Kirkland, Washington, and co-author of *Juicing for Life*. Dark-colored berries such as cherries, blackberries, and blueberries contain anthocyanins and proanthocyanidins, pigments that, according to Calbom, tone and strengthen the walls of hemorrhoidal veins, which can minimize pain and swelling.

To maximize the therapeutic benefits of these pigments, Calbom suggests drinking 4 ounces of dark berry juice diluted with 4 ounces of apple juice at least once a day.

Slash your coffee drinking. Coffee beans contain oils that you can't digest. The oils irritate the skin surrounding the anus when they are excreted from the body. Simply limiting yourself to one or two 6-ounce cups of coffee daily may be enough to prevent or relieve anal itching, says Scott Goldstein, M.D., a colon and rectal surgeon at Thomas Jefferson University Hospital in Philadelphia.

Tame a rebel with a gauze. Place a thin strip of gauze or cotton up against the anal opening to absorb excessive sweat and mucus and to prevent rashes and itching, says Dr. Orkin.

Make like a boxer. Loose cotton underwear is a better choice than clinging nylon or polyester because it absorbs moisture better and allows more air to pass through, keeping your bottom dry, says Dr. Orkin.

Sock it to pinworms. Pinworms generally infect young children, but other family members can attract the unwanted attention of these pests, which come out at night and cause infernal anal itching. Your doctor can prescribe an oral antiparasitic medication to relieve the problem, but you also should thoroughly wash all bedding in hot water to prevent a recurrence.

Check your medications. Some drugs can cause anal itching. Antibiotics, for example, often destroy harmless bacteria in the anus that fight off itchy yeast infections. Ask your doctor if your medications may be causing your problem.

Blow your itch away. Using a hair dryer set on low for 20 to 30 seconds after bathing or swimming is a good way to gently but thoroughly dry your bottom and prevent itching. One precaution: If you feel your skin burning, either the dryer is set too high or it is too close.

Bare your bottom to the sun. "The sun's ultraviolet light can help prevent and relieve itching and other irritations in the anal area and dry the skin. Nude sunbathing is a great way to get some of that sunlight into areas of your backside that are usually left in the dark," says Eric G. Anderson, M.D., a family practice physician in La Jolla, California. As with more modest forms of sun worshipping, you should always apply a sunscreen to exposed skin and build up your time in the sun gradually.

Don't worry. Believe it or not, if you feel anxious or are under a lot of stress, you may develop an itchy anus. Relieving your stress through yoga, progressive relaxation, or exercise might end your scratching.

In his book *Healing Visualizations*, New York City psychiatrist Gerald Epstein, M.D., suggests this remedy for hemorrhoids: Close your eyes, breathe out three times, and imagine that your hemorrhoids are puckering up like an old purse. Picture them shriveling and disappearing as the walls of the anus become pink and smooth. Dr. Epstein says to practice this imagery for 1 to 2 minutes of

When to See a Doctor

- You notice bleeding from your rectum.
- You feel a lump in the rectal area.
- You have diabetes.
- You are taking steroids.
- Your children complain of anal itching.

every waking hour, for up to 21 days, until the hemorrhoids fade.

Wash, don't wipe. Good hygiene is crucial to preventing anal itching. If possible, after each bowel movement wash your anus with a soft cloth dipped in warm water and mild soap. Rinse and pat dry; don't rub.

Go for the plain paper. "You should stick to plain, two-ply soft toilet paper and avoid fancy stuff," Dr. Goldstein says. "You don't want anything like perfumes in those papers that may irritate the skin."

Soothe painful hemorrhoids with a good soak. Says Greenwich, Connecticut, aromatherapist Judith Jackson, author of *Scentual Touch: A Personal Guide to Aromatherapy*: Add 20 drops each of lavender and juniper essential oils to a hot, shallow bath, mixing the bathwater with your hand to make sure the oils are well-dispersed. Then soak for 10 minutes.

Increase your fiber intake. A high-fiber diet is the key to preventing or treating hemorrhoids, says Michael A. Klaper, M.D., a nutritional medicine specialist in Pompano Beach, Florida, and director of the Institute of Nutritional Education and Research in Manhattan Beach, California. Hard, constipated stool means you need to push harder to defecate, he explains, and when you push hard, your hemorrhoidal veins bulge. Fiber makes your stool soft, putting less pressure on the veins. Dr. Klaper suggests trying to consume at least 30 grams of fiber each day by eating at least five servings of fresh fruits and vegetables and more whole grains, beans, and bran products.

Turn to St. John's wort. It can help relieve the itching and burning of hemorrhoids, says Barre, Vermont, herbalist Rosemary Gladstar, author of *Herbal Healing for Women*. Health food stores carry salves made with this herb; Gladstar says to follow the directions on the label of the product you choose.

Try some witch hazel. Gladstar says to moisten cotton cloths with witch hazel extract and apply the cloths as compresses, leaving them on for 15 to 20 minutes twice a day. Keep both the witch hazel extract and the cloths in the refrigerator, she suggests; they'll retain their freshness and feel cool and soothing when you use them.

Opt for a strong, cold black tea compress. It is very soothing to hemorrhoids, says Agatha Thrash, M.D., a medical pathologist and cofounder and codirector of Uchee Pines Institute, a natural healing center in Seale, Alabama. She suggests holding the compress against the hemorrhoids for several minutes.

Back Pain

Eight out of 10 people experience back problems sometime in their lives. And when they feel back pain, it's often in the lower back because it gets so much use. This part of the spine links your upper body (chest and arms) to your lower body (pelvis and legs). It lets you turn to greet a friend or stoop to kiss a baby, and it gives you strength to stand, walk, or lift a box. Most lower-back problems, though painful, are not caused by serious medical conditions. Poor muscle tone and improper movement often are the culprits.

Whatever the cause, there are lots of ways you can help yourself feel better today or prevent back pain tomorrow.

Go mobile. Resist the urge to rest in bed, especially for more than 2 to 3 days, says Steven Mandel, M.D., clinical professor of neurology at Thomas Jefferson University Hospital in Philadelphia. Studies show that light activity actually hastens healing. If you feel that you need bed rest, take it, but try walking around every few hours, even if you have a little pain, he says. A stroll around the house or yard will help strengthen muscles and keep them limber.

Until you're feeling better, though, avoid activities that may strain the lower back, such as vacuuming or gardening, says Anthony Wheeler, M.D., a neurologist in private practice in Charlotte, North Carolina.

Pack some ice. To relieve backache, reach for an ice pack, says Sheila Reid, therapy coordinator at the Spine Institute of New England in Williston, Vermont. Apply it for 5 to 10 minutes at a time.

Alternately, fill a paper cup with water, freeze it, peel back the paper, and rub the ice on sore spots, Dr. Wheeler says. Don't hold the ice on the area for more than 20 minutes and keep a thin towel between you and the ice to prevent damage to your skin.

Then try some heat. After the first couple of days, you may get more comfort from the warmth of a heating pad, bath, or shower. Try moist heat, Dr. Wheeler says. Rinse a small towel under hot water and wring it to near dry. Apply heat for up to 15 minutes at a time.

If you use a heating pad on a medium setting, be careful not to fall asleep or leave it on too long, Dr. Wheeler says. You could burn your skin.

Reach for the home stretch. As soon as you're able, add some gentle stretches to your daily routine. This will speed healing and increase flexibility, says Dr. Mandel.

Try this exercise. Lie on the floor on your back and hug your knees to your chest. Hold for 15 seconds. Relax. Repeat two times. Go to the point of stretch, not to the point of pain, Reid says.

If you can't get down on the floor, you can still stretch, Reid says. Sit in a sturdy chair with your feet flat on the floor. Lean forward from your waist, bringing your chest slowly toward your thighs. Breathe in on the way down and let the air out with a sigh as you lower yourself. Hold the stretch for 15 seconds. Do this stretch as often as you like.

When to See a Doctor

- Your pain is severe.
- It lasts more than 3 days.
- It radiates to your hips or legs.
- The pain is sudden and you've never had backache before.

Or try this standing stretch. Stand with your feet shoulder-width apart, with your hands on the small of your back. Lean backward as you breathe out, then ease off and repeat several times. This promotes a backward motion of the spine, Reid says.

Give yourself a lift. Bending and lifting incorrectly are major causes of back pain, says John E. Thomassy, D.C., a chiropractor in private practice in Virginia Beach, Virginia. "Even if you're not lifting anything, 70 percent of your body weight is above the waist." That means a 150-pound person lifts about 100 pounds every time he bends.

Don't lift with your back. The next time you reach for a suitcase in your car trunk, bend your hips and knees, keeping your back straight, Dr. Thomassy says.

Hold on tight. When you're carrying luggage, keep it close to you. The farther away you hold an object, the heavier it feels, Dr. Wheeler says. And avoid lifting loads of more than 5 to 10 pounds, he advises.

Be straight. If you're moving a box, don't pick it up and twist your body. "Never bend and twist," Dr. Thomassy says. Instead, grasp the box diagonally from the bottom, keeping it close to your body. Lift with your legs and buttock muscles while keeping your back straight. Then face squarely to where you set it down.

Please don't be seated. Sitting can actually aggravate back problems, Dr. Thomassy says. Sleeping or sitting for long periods on soft, cushy sofas or recliners can cause your back to slouch or your neck and head to be held forced forward, he says.

Get out of a slump. When you're sitting at your desk, try not to slouch, Reid cautions. Tuck a pillow or rolled towel behind your lower back for extra support. Or invest in a high-end office chair with a seat height and seat pan (the forward-back tilt of your seat) that can be adjusted to meet your needs, Reid says.

Stand safely. When you're standing for long periods of time, that, too, can aggravate back pain. Vary your position, Reid says. While standing, keep one foot on a low stool. Or keep a taller stool nearby so you can sometimes sit while you work, Dr. Wheeler suggests. And run errands during off-peak hours so you won't have to spend as much time standing in line.

Sleep right. To prevent or minimize back pain at night, keep your spine in a neutral position, Dr. Thomassy says. Don't prop your head and neck on a big pillow. Instead, choose one that keeps your head and neck in line with your upper back. "Sleep only on your side or your back, but never on your stomach," he says. Sleeping on your stomach twists your neck and back. Also, avoid extremes in surfaces, such as saggy mattresses or bare floors. A good mattress and pillow will maintain your neck and back in the correct posture even while you sleep. Pillows between your knees or along your back or sides may provide further comfort to your back and shoulders.

Or, Dr. Wheeler says, if you're on your back, prop a pillow under your knees.

Ease into the driver's seat. To get safely into your car, lower yourself backward onto the seat, keeping your feet on the ground. Bring one leg and then the other into the car, "even if you have to use your hands to pick up your legs," Dr. Thomassy says. To get out of the car, do the opposite. If you need to, carefully support yourself on the back of the seat as you rise.

Ride in style. If you're driving or riding in the car on a long trip, use a small pillow and vary its position on your back for comfort. Take a break about every 2 hours and walk a bit. Your back will thank you for it, says Dr. Thomassy.

Bad Breath

The culprits are bacteria that live mainly in difficult-to-clean areas of the mouth such as between the teeth and on the top of the tongue. These bacteria like to feast on stagnant saliva or dying epithelial (surface) cells. As a result, they give off volatile sulfur compounds as a by-product. When the environment of the mouth becomes dry, these compounds, which smell like rotten eggs, evaporate and become airborne. Here's how to ground them for good.

Get in a scrape. Scrape that film of bacteria off your tongue with one of the spoon-shaped devices that are designed for this purpose, which are available in drugstores. Or just use a plastic spoon.

At first, you need to scrape the very back one-third of the tongue 12 to 15 times, says Jon Richter, D.M.D., Ph.D., director of the Richter Center for Breath Disorders in Philadelphia. But if you do it on a regular basis, four or five scrapes twice a day should help. To relax your tongue, grasp it with a gauze square that you hold with your fingers, and pull it out gently, rather than just sticking it out.

To reduce gagging as you scrape, breathe deeply through your nose to relax. "Scraping the tongue is the simplest approach and will produce the most dramatic short-term relief," says Dr. Richter.

Go for gargling. Gargle with a mouthwash for about 30 seconds every morning. It helps flush out those vile bacteria in a way that you might not be able to if you can't overcome gagging with a scraper. "With gargling, you're able to get quite far back. You really get to the back of the throat," says Israel Kleinberg, D.D.S., Ph.D., professor and chairman of the department of oral biology and pathology at the School of Dental Medicine, State University of New York at Stony Brook. Look for products that contain zinc (the longest acting), sodium chlorite, or other formulations that kill bacteria.

Practice the basics. If you don't clean your teeth, then you provide more of an environment for odor-causing bacteria to lodge, feed, and give off their noxious fumes, says Clifford W. Whall Jr., Ph.D., director of product evaluation for the American Dental Association. So brush your teeth at least twice a day and floss at least once a day to remove plaque and bacteria. It's also important to make room in your schedule for regular visits to your dentist for professional cleanings and checkups. This will ensure that both your breath and your oral health are at their best, says Dr. Whall.

Don't stop short. Brush for at least 2 minutes. "Most people don't brush long enough," says Dr. Whall. "You don't have to brush hard, just thoroughly." Make sure to brush the fronts and backs of your teeth, especially along your gumline. When you floss, gently scrape the sides of each tooth, pulling away from the gums.

Do right by your dentures. Dentures can absorb bad odors in the mouth, says Mel Rosenberg, Ph.D., secretary general of the International Society of Breath Odor Research and a researcher and associate professor at the Maurice and Gabriela Goldschlelger School of Dental Medicine at Tel Aviv University in Israel. Unless your dentist tells you otherwise, always soak your dentures overnight in an antiseptic solution.

Clean your dentures every day, brushing them with a commercial denture cleaner, recommends Ken Yaegaki, Ph.D., clinical professor in the department of oral biological and medical sciences at the University of British Columbia in Vancouver. If you don't have denture cleaner on hand, use toothpaste instead for 1 to 2 minutes. It's not as good, but it will help remove odor-causing bacteria, Dr. Yaegaki says.

Keep those juices flowing. If dry mouth is contributing to your bad breath, you'll need to kick your salivary glands into gear. One way to get your salivary glands going is to eat an orange or have some orange juice. The citric acid in the orange prompts the flow of saliva, says Dr. Kleinberg.

Even occasionally spritzing a little water in your mouth can help, adds Dr. Kleinberg. And be aware that although the acid in diet sodas can stimulate saliva flow, they can also erode tooth enamel. In some individuals with gum recession and exposed roots, this can result in erosion of some of the covering over the roots, causing your teeth to be sensitive to hot and cold.

Break the fast. Make sure you eat three meals a day. "Skipping meals is bad," says Dr. Richter. The very process of eating helps scrape bacteria off the tongue and stimulates the washing action of saliva. Also, as the time lengthens between meals, the mouth gets a chance to dry out, and bacteria builds up.

Body Odor

The popular notion that body odor is the smell of sweat is true . . . sort of. We actually produce two kinds of sweat: *eccrine*, a clear, odorless sweat that appears all over our bodies, performing the vital role of regulating body temperature, and *apocrine*, a thicker substance that is produced by glands in the underarm and groin areas. Apocrine sweat is a vestige of our prehistoric days and serves no apparent purpose. It, too, is odorless—until bacteria on the skin's surface act upon it. The by-product of this unholy union is what we call B.O.

"The intensity of some body odor may lead people to think that they have a serious medical problem, when in most cases they are merely the victims of bad genes or inadequate hygiene," says Selma Targovnik, M.D., staff dermatologist at Good Samaritan Medical Center in Phoenix. "Most B.O. sufferers were simply born with larger, more active apocrine glands, or else they aren't doing as good a job as they should keeping the odor-producing bacteria off their skin."

The secret to combating most body odors is to inhibit the body's production of apocrine sweat, decrease the number of bacteria acting upon that sweat, or remove the offender. Give these tips a try for success against B.O.

Wash daily with a deodorant soap. "Using an antibacterial soap like Dial or Safeguard will work well on the bacteria that are producing the odor," says Dr. Targovnik. "You don't have to scrub long or hard; the antibacterial will do all the work. Use it at least once a day, twice, if possible." If these fail, more powerful prescription soaps like pHisoHex and Hibiclens are available.

Zap it like a zit. If antibacterial soaps aren't producing results, Dr. Targovnik suggests washing the areas with an acne cleanser such as those that contain benzoyl peroxide, which has strong antibacterial properties. But be aware: Excessive use could cause drying and irritation. If these cleansers don't work, you can also try dabbing on some Neosporin or an antibacterial ointment.

Freshen up. "During the day, if you can do a quick wash of your armpits with a wet washcloth or paper towel, you can take care of some of that odorous material that has been produced as well as many of those bacteria that will produce odor in the future," says Dr. Targovnik.

Use a deodorant. "Over-the-counter underarm deodorants work fine on all odor-producing areas," says Stephen Z. Smith, M.D., a dermatologist in private practice and clinical instructor in the department of dermatology at the University of Louisville School of Medicine in Kentucky. "The deodorant should contain antibacterial metallic salts (aluminum or zinc) to kill odor-causing bacteria. Roll-ons and sticks provide better coverage and longer-lasting protection than sprays."

Try an antiperspirant. "Commercial antiperspirants slow down some of the apocrine sweat production," adds Dr. Smith. "They should contain aluminum chlorohydrate as their active ingredient and are often combined with deodorants."

Powder the offensive area. "Sprinkling some baking soda, talc, baby powder, or cornstarch under the arms or across the body will absorb and mask many of the odors produced," says R. Kenneth Landow, M.D., clinical associate professor in the department of medicine and dermatology at the University of Southern California in Los Angeles.

Get the odor out of your clothes. Wash your clothes with an odor-fighting detergent. If necessary, take a change of clothes or underwear with you to work or school.

Rub on some alcohol. "You may want to try directly applying a splash or two of some rubbing alcohol, witch hazel, or hydrogen peroxide during the day just as some extra maintenance," recommends Dr. Landow. These substances help reduce the number of odor-causing bacteria. Aim your splash where bacteria hang out—under the arms, for instance.

Avoid spicy, pungent foods. Frequent consumption of foods containing garlic, curry, and cumin can cause some overpowering odors to emanate from your pores—often up to 24 hours after consumption. Try cutting back on these spices and see if it helps.

Trim underarm and body hair. "Since men are the biggest offenders, they should follow the example of women and shave their armpits," says Dr. Targovnik. "The hairs trap a lot of the sweat and odor and provide hiding places for the bacteria."

Boils

These painful oversize pimples have less to do with personal hygiene than you might think. They're usually caused when friction (from ill-fitting undergarments or a tight shirt collar) or a scratch allows bacteria under your skin.

The bacteria, *Staphylococcus aureus*, settle in a hair follicle or an oil gland, where they are attacked by your immune system. The result is a red, pus-filled nodule. In time, the boil will be absorbed by your body or will erupt and drain.

Boils are usually harmless, but it's not a good idea to squeeze one. The natural remedies in this chapter, used with the approval of your doctor, may provide relief, according to some health professionals.

Reach for tea tree oil. It's a great natural antiseptic that speeds the healing of virtually any kind of skin irritation, says San Francisco herbalist Jeanne Rose, chairperson of the National Association for Holistic Aromatherapy and author of *Aromatherapy: Applications and Inhalations*. She suggests applying a single drop of tea tree oil directly to the boil after bathing until the boil goes away.

Bring it to a head. Here's how, according to Vasant Lad, B.A.M.S., M.A.Sc., director of the Ayurvedic Institute in Albuquerque, New Mexico: Apply a paste made from ½ teaspoon each of ginger powder and turmeric and enough warm water to mix. Rub the paste directly on the affected area, cover with gauze, and leave in place for a half-hour. Repeat as necessary until the boil breaks and begins to heal. Turmeric can stain skin and clothes, cautions Dr. Lad, so be sure to wear old garments when using this remedy. Any skin discoloration should wash off in 2 weeks, he adds.

Eat right. "Eat foods that are rich in vitamin A and zinc, because these nutrients aid in skin healing and repair and can help relieve boils," says Allan Magaziner, D.O., a nutritional medicine specialist and head of the Magaziner Medical Center in Cherry Hill, New Jersey. "Good sources of vitamin A include any fruit or vegetable that has a yellow or orange color—squash, yams, sweet potatoes, and carrots. Zinc is found in oysters, sunflower seeds, and pumpkin seeds. Vitamin A is also found in dark green leafy vegetables such as spinach and kale."

Give compresses a try. Alternating hot and cold compresses speeds the healing of a boil by increasing the flow of blood to the affected area, says Agatha Thrash, M.D., a medical pathologist and cofounder and codirector of Uchee Pines Institute, a natural healing center in Seale, Alabama. Soak a washcloth in comfortably hot water and hold it against the boil, refreshing the heat as necessary to keep the cloth hot. After 3 to 5 minutes, apply a cold compress for 30 to 60 seconds. Repeat this treatment three times daily until the boil comes to a head or goes away.

Get rid of toxins. Boils result from a buildup of toxins in the system, according to Eve Campanelli, Ph.D., a holistic family practitioner in Beverly Hills, California. To stimulate the liver and speed up the elimination of wastes, she recommends drinking a blend of 8 ounces of carrot juice, 1 ounce of beet juice, 4 ounces of celery juice, and ½ to 1 ounce of parsley juice. "A large glass each morning and a smaller glass in the afternoon is an effective and a very nutritious way to get the liver moving," says Dr. Campanelli.

Take your vitamins. To relieve a boil, take 10,000 international units of vitamin A and 15 to 20 milligrams of zinc, advises Dr. Magaziner. If you're prone to boils, keep taking these nutrients, but cut the dosage in half after the boil disappears, he says. And if boils aren't a chronic problem for you, he advises that you stop taking the supplements after the boil has cleared up.

Brittle Nails

The thickness and strength of your nails can be strongly influenced by your genes. Of course, you may not be helping matters if you use your nails as staple removers or bite at them constantly. Maybe you're exposing your nails to harsh chemicals or using too much nail polish remover, both of which deprive your nails of moisture.

The following natural remedies may help improve the strength and appearance of your nails, according to some health professionals.

Give them a soak. Brittle nails benefit from a warm fragrant oil soak, according to Greenwich, Connecticut, aromatherapist Judith Jackson, author of *Scentual Touch: A Personal Guide to Aromatherapy*. Add six drops of lavender, six drops of bay, and six drops of sandalwood essential oils to 6 ounces of warm sesame oil or soy oil, suggests Jackson. Soak for 15 minutes once or twice a week.

Eat your fish. Cold-water fish such as salmon, mackerel, and herring are rich in omega-3 fatty acids, which can strengthen nails, advises Julian Whitaker, M.D., founder and president of the Whitaker Wellness Center in Newport Beach, California. He also recommends cauliflower, soybeans, peanuts, walnuts, and lentils, which are all rich in biotin, a B vitamin that he says can prevent the splitting and cracking that are associated with brittle nails.

Reach for flaxseed oil. It's got essential fatty acids that strengthen nails, says Dr. Whitaker. It comes in capsule or liquid form. Follow the dosage recommendations on the label. Flaxseed oil is available in health food stores.

Practice a little yoga. Brittle nails are sometimes the result of bad digestion and may be helped with a daily exercise called the stomach lift, says Stephen A. Nezezon, M.D., yoga teacher and staff physician at the Himalayan International Institute of Yoga Science and Philosophy in Honesdale, Pennsylvania.

Start by standing with your feet about 2 feet apart. Keep your back straight and bend forward slightly at the waist. Place your left palm on your left thigh, just above the knee, and your right palm in the same place on your right thigh. Breathe out all the way, then bend your neck forward so that your chin tucks into your throat.

Without breathing, suck in your stomach muscles as if you were trying to touch your belly button to your backbone. Hold this as long as possible, then relax and breathe. Stand up straight. Repeat this three times.

Because of its impact on the circulatory system, Dr. Nezezon says not to do this exercise during menstruation or pregnancy, after surgery, if you are bleeding, or if you have heart disease or high blood pressure.

Bruises

We've all had our share of bruises. It takes just one good, swift blow, and the blood vessels beneath your skin rupture, spilling blood into the surrounding tissues and creating the colorful palette of blacks, blues, purples, yellows, and greens we know as a bruise. For the bruise to heal, the body must reabsorb all of that spilled blood, which, depending on the extent of the damage, could take days or even weeks.

If you're prone to bruising, basic first-aid treatment can help you heal. Apply an ice pack, wrapped in a towel, on and off for the first 24 hours, followed by warm compresses the next day. If you really want to give bruises the old heave-ho and make yourself less "bruisable" in the future, try these suggestions.

Chase the blues away with vitamin K. Research shows that applying vitamin K topically can fade away bruises, says longtime vitamin K investigator Melvin L. Elson, M.D., medical director of the Dermatology Center in Nashville, co-author of *The Good Look Book*, and editor of *Evaluation and Treatment of the Aging Face.*

71

Moreover, vitamin K strengthens blood vessel walls, so it also makes you less prone to bruising, explains Dr. Elson, who has developed a 1 percent cream called Vitamin K Clarifying Cream. The cream is available only through a physician, so if you'd like to try some "bruise guard," check with your doctor.

Can you also ward off bruises by eating more vitamin K–rich foods such as green, leafy vegetables, fruits, seeds, and dairy products? "There's no absolute proof, but studies seem to indicate that you can," says Dr. Elson. Even though getting plenty of vitamin K— the Daily Value is 80 micrograms—may be helpful, when you have a bruise or an area prone to bruising, you want large doses of vitamin K right where you need them, and the best way to get them there is topically, says Dr. Elson.

Get help from C. Vitamin C, the nutrient abundant in citrus fruits and broccoli, may also help strengthen the collagen (skin tissue) around your blood vessels and help battle bruises.

"There is some evidence that supplemental vitamin C at the level of 500 to 1,000 milligrams per day is quite useful against the bruising of old age," says Sheldon Pinnell, M.D., chief of dermatology at Duke University Medical Center in Durham, North Carolina.

For even better results, try a topical form of vitamin C, says Dr. Pinnell, who has developed a 10 percent vitamin C lotion called Cellex-C. "By using the lotion, you get 20 to 40 times the level of vitamin C that you could achieve by ingesting the vitamin."

Cellex-C is available without a prescription from dermatologists, plastic surgeons, and licensed aestheticians (full-service beauty salon operators).

Eat Your Bioflavonoids

Some researchers believe that bioflavonoids—chemical compounds related to vitamin C and found in fruits and vegetables—may help prevent bruises. Eating plenty of oranges and other citrus fruits can boost your level of rutin, a bioflavonoid that was singled out by researchers in the 1950s as one that could help strengthen fragile capillaries and minimize the bruising that often accompanies this condition.

"It's important to remember that although this compound may prevent some bruises from occurring, it isn't good for the treatment of a bruise after it has happened," says Varro E. Tyler, Ph.D., professor of pharmacognosy at Purdue University School of Pharmacy in West Lafayette, Indiana.

Rutin is also found in buckwheat. So here's a good excuse to enjoy a hearty breakfast of buckwheat pancakes.

Let zinc lend a helping hand. Although its role in bruise healing is not as well-researched or defined as those of vitamins C and K, zinc plays a role in wound healing and may help with bruises.

You can get your Daily Value of zinc (15 milligrams) by filling your plate with shellfish and other seafood as well as with whole grains and lean meats. In fact, just one steamed oyster contains 12.7 milligrams.

Canker Sores

Canker sores lie on the inner lining of your lips and cheeks or on the base of your tongue, the floor of your mouth, or your soft palate. These painful critters are yellowish gray or white with red borders. They're tiny, round, and appear individually or in bunches. They're not contagious and normally heal within 7 to 14 days. But they can turn the simple pleasures of eating, talking, and even brushing your teeth into harrowing experiences.

Fortunately, there are dietary and other natural measures that can keep these little buggers out of your mouth. Start by eliminating the top canker sore triggers from your diet, such as chocolate, nuts, tomatoes, green peppers, strawberries, and oranges and other citrus fruits. Try to avoid eating sharp-edged corn chips and pretzels, because they can irritate and injure the lining of your mouth and produce an ulcer.

After you've eliminated the troublemakers, you can reintroduce each of these foods into your diet one at a time every 2 to 3 days to determine which is the source of the trouble. Canker sores can also be caused by food sensitivities to wheat products. See your doctor to determine whether food allergies are causing your problem. Otherwise, try these remedies.

Zap canker sores with licorice. What you want is deglycyrrhizinated licorice (DGL), not the black, stringy stuff kids eat. "DGL has anti-inflammatory properties. It speeds the healing process and soothes the discomfort of canker sores," says Michael Traub, N.D., a naturopathic doctor and director of the integrated residency program at North Hawaii Community Hospital in Kamuela.

To begin the healing process, take two 200-milligram tablets 20 minutes before meals, says Dr. Traub, or chew one or two tablets two or three times a day. While chewing, use your tongue to position the tablet residue on the sore to promote even speedier healing. Use DGL, available at health food stores, until the sore heals.

In addition, you can empty the powder from a capsule into ½ cup of lukewarm water, dissolve the DGL, and swish the solution around in your mouth, says Dr. Traub. Repeat this at least two or three times a day until the sore has healed.

Cover your bases with a multivitamin. Deficiencies of some B vitamins and minerals seem prevalent among people with canker sores. When the deficiencies are corrected, the sores often show improvement or complete remission.

"Low levels of some B vitamins can cause swelling of the tongue and canker sores. If you're not getting enough zinc, you won't heal as quickly from small injuries like biting the inside of your mouth. And without enough folic acid and iron, you won't maintain the necessary rapid cell division that you need to keep the lining of your mouth healthy," says Jennifer Brett, N.D., a naturopathic doctor at the Wilton Naturopathic Center in Stratford, Connecticut.

A high-potency multivitamin should give you the nutrients that are necessary to prevent recurrent canker sores, says Dr. Brett. Take 500 to 1,000 micrograms of vitamin B_{12}, 10 milligrams of iron, 800 micrograms of folic acid, and 15 to 20 milligrams of zinc, she says. If your multivitamin doesn't include all you need, simply add separate supplements to make up the difference.

Seek more solutions from C and thiamin. If your canker sores are a result of food allergies, take 1,000 to 1,200 milligrams of buffered vitamin C daily to help reduce the level of histamines in your body, says Dr. Brett. Histamines are the immune system chemicals that cause inflammation and irritation. To enhance the effectiveness of the vitamin C, take 1,000 milligrams of quercetin or 100 milligrams of grape seed extract daily as a preventive, she says. These are both bioflavonoids, compounds that inhibit histamine release, reduce inflammation, and speed healing.

Other research shows that a deficiency of thiamin can lead to recurrent mouth ulcers. Dr. Brett recommends taking 100 milligrams of thiamin daily as a preventive.

Cold Sores

A tingling sensation outside your mouth or above your lips is usually the telltale sign. Within 2 to 3 days, a painful, fluid-filled blister appears. It swells, ruptures, and oozes fluid that forms a yellow crust. Eventually, it peels off and reveals new skin underneath. The blister usually lasts 7 to 10 days, but while it's in full view, you may be tempted to go into hiding or cover your mouth with your hands until the unsightly sore disappears.

What causes cold sores, commonly called fever blisters, is herpes simplex virus type 1. About 90 percent of all people are infected with it, and if you get a sore once, you'll get another. If you change your diet and take some other natural measures, you might be able to shorten the time that these sores stay on your mouth and lips.

Heal them with lysine. This amino acid inhibits the replication of herpes simplex. Research suggests that a diet high in lysine and low in arginine can prevent the virus from multiplying. Although it relies on arginine to thrive, the virus can't distinguish between lysine and arginine, so it's easily tricked into attaching itself to the lysine. But unlike arginine, lysine blocks the steps the virus must take to replicate.

To keep lysine levels high, take 500 to 1,500 milligrams daily at the first sign of symptoms, says Jennifer Brett, N.D., a naturopathic doctor at the Wilton Naturopathic Center in Stratford, Connecticut. Continue with that dosage until symptoms disappear.

If you're having an outbreak, take 3,000 milligrams of lysine daily until the lesions go away.

Zap them with vitamin C and bioflavonoids. These supplements boost your immune system by stimulating production of white blood cells, the infection fighters in your body. The blisters will heal faster as a result, says Dr. Brett.

Bioflavonoids, chemical compounds related to vitamin C, can help reduce the inflammation and pain that's associated with cold sores, says Dr. Brett. You can buy a formula that includes both or take each as a separate supplement.

To prevent cold sores, take 1,000 milligrams of vitamin C with bioflavonoids daily, Dr. Brett advises. To speed the healing of existing sores, she recommends taking 3,000 milligrams of vitamin C daily in divided doses and 1,000 milligrams daily of quercetin, a commonly used bioflavonoid.

Zinc 'em, too. Upping your intake of zinc can also reduce the frequency, duration, and severity of cold sore outbreaks. This mineral has been shown in test-tube studies to block the reproduction of the virus.

During a cold sore outbreak, take 50 milligrams a day of zinc in divided doses with food, says Michael Traub, N.D., a naturopathic doctor and director of the integrated residency program at North Hawaii Community Hospital in Kamuela. As a preventive, take 20 milligrams a day. Also, since zinc supplementation can lead to copper deficiency, you should take 1 to 2 milligrams of copper for every 25 milligrams of zinc you take, says Dr. Traub. Don't exceed 2 milligrams of copper daily, however.

Call on a pair of antiviral herbs. Medicinal herbs such as echinacea and St. John's wort can also speed healing, lessen the severity, and shorten the duration of cold sores, says Dr. Traub.

Dr. Traub recommends taking one 300-milligram capsule of echinacea four times a day during a cold sore outbreak. For prevention, take one 300-milligram capsule daily during times of stress or as soon as you feel a cold sore coming on, he says. During an outbreak, take one 300-milligram capsule of St. John's wort daily; buy the standardized extract that contains 0.3 percent hypericin.

Constipation

We all know when we're constipated, but we might not know what's causing the problem. "A lot of constipation just comes down to diet, water, and exercise," says Melissa Metcalfe, N.D., a naturopathic doctor in Los Angeles.

Other causes include stress, dehydration, hemorrhoids, or anal fissures. A colon with weak muscle tone can also cause constipation.

"If there aren't serious underlying causes, the cure is pretty simple," says Dr. Metcalfe. That's where these remedies can help.

Drink up. Your first self-treatment should be water. It adds soft bulk to stools. It's also required by the cells of the colon to lubricate the stool's passage, says Dr. Metcalfe. "If dehydration is your only problem, you can be having a normal bowel movement in less than 24 hours," she says.

At the very least, you should drink eight full 8-ounce glasses of water a day, she says. If you're physically active or drink coffee and other caffeinated beverages that make you urinate often, you should drink 12 glasses a day to compensate for that dehydration. "I tell patients to put 2 liters of water in the fridge and make sure it is gone at the end of the day."

If you don't like the taste of tap water, buy bottled water or some type of filtering system, she suggests.

Fill up with fiber. Dietary fiber absorbs water and makes stools fuller and easier to pass. The result is faster transit time through the intestines.

Both soluble and insoluble fiber absorb water. Soluble fiber essentially turns into a kind of gel in your intestine. Good food sources include prunes, apples, kidney beans and other legumes, and oats.

For insoluble fiber, turn to bran, wheat, and vegetables like celery, carrots, and spinach. You should get 25 grams of total fiber a day.

Although it's best to get your fiber from food sources, you can also take a supplement when your meals aren't supplying enough. Dr. Metcalfe recommends 2 tablespoons daily of a fiber/nutritional supplement that contains psyllium. You can also add 2 tablespoons of flaxseed to yogurt or make a "smoothie" with blended yogurt, fruit, and flaxseed.

Move to have movement. To get things moving down below, get off your duff, says Pamela Taylor, N.D., a naturopathic doctor in Moline, Illinois.

Two layers of muscles around the small intestine work together in a process called peristalsis, the wavelike contraction that moves digested food and waste products through the gastrointestinal system. People who are sedentary, particularly if they're older, often lack muscle tone in the abdominal area.

"Exercise can tone abdominal muscles, massage the abdominal organs, and increase blood flow to the area. All of that can help restore good bowel function," says Dr. Taylor.

When to See a Doctor

- You are constipated frequently.
- Every attempt at a bowel movement involves a lot of pain.

See about senna. If diet and lifestyle changes don't do the trick, as a last resort you can try senna, a strong-acting herb that stimulates peristalsis, says Dr. Metcalfe. Its active ingredient, a chemical called anthraquinone, is responsible for this effect.

You might want to use senna as a one-time option, suggests Kristin Stiles, N.D., a naturopathic doctor at the Complementary Medicine and Healing Arts Center in Vestal, New York. It's not safe to use for long-term, chronic constipation. If you take senna repeatedly, your bowel may lose the ability to function on its own.

Dr. Metcalfe recommends that you purchase senna tea bags at a health food store and start off with no more than 1 cup of senna tea each morning. "Senna is probably going to cause some cramping at first. It really increases peristalsis quickly, so you want to start off slowly with it," she cautions.

Senna works well in combination with psyllium. Although both laxatives increase the frequency of bowel movements, the combination provides more moisture in stools and more relief.

Because senna is a powerful herb that has some risks, you should seek the advice of a naturopathic physician before taking it. Women who are pregnant or breastfeeding should not take senna.

Coughing

Most people cough at least once or twice an hour. It's a natural reflex that clears the throat and helps keep irritants out of the lungs. But when coughing keeps you awake at night, grows so persistent that you are physically tired, or becomes so annoying that no one can stand being around you, it's not normal.

Bouts of coughing are usually the result of an infection caused by a cold or flu. Coughs can also be caused by stomach acids creeping into the esophagus, by inhaling irritants such as cigarette smoke, or by breathing cold, dry air.

Before treating your cough, you need to figure out whether you *should* treat it. There are two kinds of coughs. First, there's a productive cough. That's the kind that brings up phlegm so that you can spit it out. You want to get the phlegm out. So that kind of cough is a good cough. If possible, let it run its course.

A dry, hacking cough doesn't bring up phlegm. All it does is irritate your throat, making you cough some more. If you have a dry cough, here's how to muzzle it.

Take your medicine. There are a number of over-the-counter cough suppressants that will quickly calm a dry, hacking cough. You don't need to root through name brands. According to the American Academy of Otolaryngology, the generic brands are just as effective. Just be sure that you get the right active ingredient.

Cough suppressants usually contain one of four ingredients: codeine, dextromethorphan, diphenhydramine, or guaifenesin. Codeine is great at suppressing coughs, but it also can upset the stomach and make you constipated. A suppressant containing dextromethorphan is probably the better choice. It suppresses the nerve signals that tell your body to cough, but without the side effects caused by codeine.

Diphenhydramine is an antihistamine that can treat coughs but also will make you drowsy. Guaifenesin is an expectorant that is supposed to loosen up mucus. Though approved by the Food and Drug Administration, clinical trials haven't proved its effectiveness. Drinking lots of fluids (water, juice, tea) will make your cough more productive, regardless of whether you are taking an expectorant.

Swallow a soothing potion. Swallowing a mixture of honey, lemon juice, and ground red pepper can soothe a cough and sore throat, says Elson Haas, M.D., director of the Preventive Medical Center of Marin in San Rafael, California. The honey coats the throat, soothing the pain. The lemon is an astringent, which reduces inflammation and also clobbers germs with vitamin C. The ground red pepper brings circulation to the area, which speeds healing. It also is rich in vitamin A.

To make the potion, pour ¾ teaspoon of honey into a tablespoon and then fill the rest with lemon juice. Sprinkle the red pepper on top. You can take it four times a day, Dr. Haas says.

Rub it the right way. Menthol, a common ingredient in some over-the-counter cough drops, is the principal component of the essential oil derived from peppermint. One study found that using menthol as a chest rub reduced coughs within 30 minutes.

Raise your head. If you usually cough only at night, you might be experiencing a condition called gastroesophageal reflux, in which stomach acids creep upward into the esophagus. The American Academy of Otolaryngology recommends elevating the head of your bed 6 to 8 inches to keep the acids from creeping upstream.

Depression

When low spirits turn into a never-ending state of sadness, you may have depression. While you may not be able to tell the difference between feeling blue and being depressed, a doctor usually can.

In fact, a diagnosis of depression needs to be made by a doctor. There are many possible signs, ranging from sleeplessness and irritability to feelings of guilt or thoughts of suicide. Whether or not you have these symptoms, though, you should seek professional help if you have a blue mood that lasts more than 2 weeks.

Many doctors prescribe medication for depression, and if you're already taking medication, you shouldn't take supplements without talking to your doctor. Often, dietary and lifestyle changes can help lift your mood, says C. Norman Shealy, M.D., Ph.D., founder of the American Holistic Medical Association and director of the Shealy Institute, a holistic and alternative medicine clinic in Springfield, Missouri. In fact, just 20 minutes of aerobic exercise 5 days a week can put that pep back in your step, says Dr. Shealy.

Studies show that any kind of exercise prompts the release of mood-enhancing brain chemicals called endorphins that help restore your sense of well-being. Also, if you avoid caffeine, alcohol, sugar, and refined carbohydrates (found in cakes and white bread, for instance), you'll prevent brain chemical imbalances that are known to cause depression.

Here are some natural antidepressant supplements that might be helpful.

Try B and C. The most common deficiencies in people who are depressed are the B-complex vitamins and vitamin C, says Dr. Shealy.

The B vitamins help energize brain cells and manufacture important chemicals to keep your moods high. Vitamin B_6 plays a starring role in the making of serotonin, a brain chemical that has a direct impact on your moods, emotions, appetite, and sleep patterns. Too little serotonin, and you'll walk around feeling down in the dumps. A folate (folic acid) deficiency is often marked by depression. Low vitamin B_{12} levels are common in elderly people with depression, and folate and B_{12} can work together to boost low spirits, says Dr. Shealy. Vitamin B_{12} also helps metabolize other mood-elevating brain chemicals and keep nerve tissue healthy.

Another vitamin important for maintaining high spirits is vitamin C. Low levels can leave you feeling gloomy, says Ray Sahelian, M.D., a physician in Marina del Rey, California, and author of The New Memory Boosters: Natural Supplements That Enhance Your Mind, Memory, and Mood. Vitamin C helps manufacture serotonin and two other essential brain-related chemicals that lift your mood, keep you alert, and sustain your sex drive.

For mild to moderate depression, you may want to take a high-potency multivitamin/mineral supplement daily after talking to your doctor, says Dr. Shealy. He also suggests 100 milligrams each of thiamin, riboflavin, niacin, and B_6, along with 400 micrograms of folate, 100 micrograms of B_{12}, and 2,000 milligrams of vitamin C in divided doses daily.

Get help from St. John. St. John's wort is the quintessential herb of choice for mild to moderate depression. In fact, it is one of the most researched natural antidepressants around. The herb's active ingredients work in unison to raise serotonin levels in the brain, says Jennifer Brett, N.D., a naturopathic doctor at the Wilton Naturopathic Center in Stratford, Connecticut.

Studies show that St. John's wort is just as effective for mild to moderate depression as the widely prescribed antidepressant drugs imipramine (Tofranil), fluoxetine (Prozac), sertraline (Zoloft), and paroxetine (Paxil), says Dr. Shealy.

The advantage of St. John's wort over the prescription antidepressants is that it's associated with very few side effects. Some people do get mild stomach irritation, and others have reported sun sensitivity and insomnia. If you are pregnant, check with your doctor before taking this or any other supplement. If you are already taking antidepressant medication, you should also talk to your doctor before taking St. John's wort.

Dr. Shealy suggests taking one 300-milligram tablet or capsule three times a day with meals if you have mild to moderate depression. For maximum effectiveness, buy a standardized extract containing 0.3 percent hypericin, he says. If you don't feel better after 4 to 6 weeks, it's unlikely to help, he adds.

Let ginkgo do some good. Although it's not as strong as St. John's wort, ginkgo can be used as a mild antidepressant. Ginkgo greatly improves blood flow, mental alertness, and memory, and—as a by-product—relieves depression, says Dr. Sahelian. "Poor blood circulation to the brain can cause the brain to malfunction, which can lead to imbalances in serotonin levels and other neurotransmitters that regulate moods and emotional stability."

If you're over age 50 and have mild to moderate depression, take one 40-milligram capsule of ginkgo three times a day, says Dr. Shealy. Choose capsules or tablets that contain 24 percent ginkgoflavoglycosides for maximum strength.

Go for brain chemicals in a pill. Another supplement that might have the edge over antidepressant prescription drugs is 5-HTP. This is a natural compound produced by the body from tryptophan, an amino acid found in many foods. It's also a precursor of serotonin, which means that more serotonin is produced when 5-HTP is present.

When you take 5-HTP in supplement form, it's absorbed in your gastrointestinal tract and then journeys to your brain, where it's converted into serotonin, says Dr. Sahelian.

If you've been diagnosed with depression and you have a doctor's approval, you can take 50 milligrams of 5-HTP late in the evening, says Dr. Sahelian. But he doesn't advise taking larger amounts. Any dosage over 50 milligrams can cause vivid dreams, nightmares, and nausea, Dr. Sahelian points out.

Dermatitis

Dermatitis is simply your immune system flashing its message—"I'm irritated"—on your skin in the form of an itchy red rash. And it doesn't take much to irritate some folks' skin. Culprits include things such as nickel and latex and even certain foods. And such outbursts occur fairly often: 10 percent of all children suffer from dermatitis at one time or another.

Doctors are now aware, however, that immune system irritation and allergy are not the only causes of dermatitis. In rare cases, vitamin and mineral deficiencies can also help launch dermatological tirades. If you deplete your body of vitamin A, biotin, other B vitamins, vitamin E, or zinc, it won't be long before a skin rash appears.

"We have known for years that minor deficiencies of certain vitamins and minerals could produce skin, hair, and nail problems in both children and adults," says Wilma Bergfeld, M.D., dermatologist and director of the Section of Dermatopathology (the study of the causes and effects of skin diseases and abnormalities) and Dermatological Research at the Cleveland Clinic. "What's far less clear is just how they cause them."

Here's how to get relief, say the experts.

Zero in on zinc. Perhaps the best-understood deficiency-dermatitis connection is the link to zinc. Imagine your roof without shingles to protect against the elements and you get a picture of your skin without zinc.

If you take in less than the Daily Value of 15 milligrams of zinc for a few weeks, the shingles of your skin—your top layer of skin cells—begin to dissolve, says Dr. Bergfeld. Without this protective layer, your skin becomes rough and crusted, opening up opportunities for bacteria, yeast, and other infections to take hold, she says.

"In a zinc deficiency, your skin simply does not perform the normal barrier function that it otherwise would," says Thomas Helm, M.D., assistant clinical professor of dermatology at the State University of New York at Buffalo and director of the Buffalo Medical Group. As a result, zinc deficiency can cause dermatitis around the mouths and rectums of young children. Such deficiencies aren't exactly common, but they occur more frequently than other nutrient-related skin problems, says Jon Hanifin, M.D., professor of dermatology at Oregon Health Sciences University in Portland.

Other people who are most susceptible to this kind of dermatitis: those with irritable bowel syndrome, those undergoing chemotherapy, alcohol-dependent people, and some moms-to-be. "In all of these cases, their zinc levels may actually go below the normal range even if they are eating enough zinc," says Dr. Helm. "It's just not being absorbed properly."

Fortunately, alleviating problems caused by a zinc deficiency is as simple as adding more zinc to your diet; you should aim for 15 milligrams a day. Even when there is a problem with zinc absorption, zinc deficiency can usually be overcome by increasing dietary zinc, Dr. Helm says.

"When zinc replacement is given, most of these rashes clear right up," agrees Dr. Bergfeld.

Give vitamin E a go. Some clinical reports seem to show vitamin E's effectiveness against some kinds of dermatitis.

Commander Patrick Olson, M.D., an epidemiologist and preventive medicine specialist at the Naval Medical

Common Food Culprits

Although rare, foods may cause dermatitis. Avoid these, which are more likely than others to do so.

Consider your moo. Milk can occasionally worsen atopic dermatitis in allergic children, says Jon Hanifin, M.D., professor of dermatology at Oregon Health Sciences University in Portland. "This allergy to milk and dairy products seems to subside as the individuals grow older," he says.

If you want to eliminate milk products from your diet, read food labels carefully. Milk can appear as an ingredient where you least expect it, says Dr. Hanifin.

Go easy on the eggs. During a Japanese study of 27 people with dermatitis, researchers found that 11 had outbreaks within 2 hours of eating eggs. If you think eggs are causing your dermatitis or eczema, avoid them, and when your skin is clear, test yourself by eating eggs again. If your dermatitis returns, avoid eggs, says Dr. Hanifin.

Say good-bye to wheat. Gluten, an ingredient in wheat, gives some people itchy red rashes on the arms, the legs, and sometimes the scalp. "It's very hard to avoid wheat products," says Stephen Schleicher, M.D., codirector of the Dermatology Center in Philadelphia. Fortunately, more and more companies are making gluten-free products.

Center in San Diego, theorizes that the antioxidant action of vitamin E prevents damage from free radicals. In this case, the damage is manifested as dermatitis. Free radicals, normal by-products of cell life, are unstable molecules that damage cells. Antioxidants neutralize free radicals and protect healthy molecules from harm.

While the Daily Value for vitamin E is only 30 international units, doses of up to 400 international units daily

(Gluten is also found in rye, barley, and oats, but in much smaller amounts.)

Shy away from shellfish. Shrimp and squid provoke dermatitis in some people. Don't be surprised if lobster, clams, mussels, and other shellfish also bring on the itchies, experts say. These often contain the same dermatitis-causing chemicals.

Search out soy. This inexpensive protein source is another trigger for atopic dermatitis in some people, says Dr. Hanifin.

Note those nuts. Peanuts round out the list of foods that most often cause dermatitis or eczema, says Dr. Hanifin.

Go fishing for fish oil. Some doctors have reported less itching and scaling in people with eczema after they took fish oil capsules containing omega-3 fatty acids. Fatty acids may help regulate inflammation and the immune response responsible for dermatitis in some. The recommended dose is 5 grams twice daily, according to Melvyn Werbach, M.D., author of *Healing through Nutrition*, but it's important to check with your doctor before taking these supplements. You can also try eating more fatty fish such as salmon, sardines, and tuna.

are considered safe. "It's just a theory, but since vitamin E seems completely benign at these doses, there's no reason why this area shouldn't be explored further," says Dr. Olson.

Turn to vitamin C for help. It's no secret that a vitamin C deficiency can damage gums and skin. And at least one study showed that taking supplements helps people with severe eczema, according to Melvyn Werbach, M.D., author of *Healing through Nutrition*. (Eczema is a type of dermatitis characterized by weeping breaks in the skin that eventually form scales.) Dr. Werbach recommends taking 3,500 to 5,000 milligrams of vitamin C each day for 3 months. This is a lot of vitamin C, as some people experience diarrhea from only 1,200 milligrams. If you'd like to try this treatment, you should discuss it with your physician.

Most dermatologists don't suggest vitamin C for dermatitis, but there are reasons that it might work, says Dr. Helm. For one thing, doctors are just learning that vitamin C seems to protect the skin from sun damage. Vitamin C speeds wound healing and prevents ultraviolet-induced free radical damage to the skin. Studies show decreased photoaging and susceptibility to sunburn in animals given vitamin C supplementation, Dr. Helm reports. "It's not unreasonable to suspect that vitamin C can help the skin stay healthy when exposed to harmful stresses other than ultraviolet light," he says.

Diarrhea

For most people, diarrhea is not a serious problem but rather an awkward, embarrassing dilemma for a day or two. Usually, it goes away on its own, unless it is a symptom of a more serious problem such as food poisoning, Crohn's disease, ulcerative colitis, or an adverse drug reaction.

If you try some remedies and use the supplements that doctors recommend, they should start to work in 24 to 48 hours.

One thing you have to be concerned about is the loss of fluids. You may not feel like drinking when your stomach is doing somersaults, but it's necessary. You should always try to sip water to avoid dehydration, says Kristin Stiles, N.D., a naturopathic doctor at the Complementary Medicine and Healing Arts Center in Vestal, New York.

Whenever you lose fluids and don't replace them, you also lose minerals that regulate many of the body's essential processes, such as blood pressure, heart rate, and muscle movements. Sports drinks are perfect for anyone with diarrhea. Sip at least 4 ounces every hour for as long as the diarrhea lasts, says Dr. Stiles. And follow these other tips.

Seek help from herbals. If your diarrhea is due to bacteria or some type of food poisoning, goldenseal and garlic can help. Both have antibacterial properties. Take 100 to 250 milligrams of goldenseal or 200 to 400 milligrams of garlic three times a day until your diarrhea subsides, recommends Dr. Stiles.

When your digestive system is trying to get rid of the contents of your stomach and intestines, there's a lot of inner activity called peristaltic movement, which sometimes causes cramping. Plus, you may get gas because the material in your intestines is starting to ferment, says Pamela Taylor, N.D., a naturopathic doctor in Moline, Illinois. To help alleviate spasms in the gastrointestinal tract, try taking a capsule or two of ginger. Dr. Taylor recommends a dosage of 200 to 400 milligrams.

Another herb that's good for relieving intestinal spasms is valerian. "It relieves stomach cramping and reduces the formation of gas," says Dr. Stiles. She recommends taking a 100- to 300-milligram capsule of valerian twice a day.

When to See a Doctor

- Your diarrhea lasts for more than 3 to 4 days.
- There is blood in the stool.
- You feel dehydrated and very weak.
- There is localized pain or fever.
- An infant or elderly adult has diarrhea that lasts more than 12 to 24 hours.

Look to glutamine for GI health. With severe diarrhea or a bout that lasts a few days, the intestines may remain inflamed, says Dr. Stiles. Try glutamine, an amino acid supplement. It encourages the quick turnover of cells along the wall of the stomach and the small intestine, she says, and makes the body heal a bit faster.

"While you're healing, I would recommend 500 milligrams of glutamine three times a day," suggests Dr. Stiles. Continue this dosage for about 2 weeks or until you have no more discomfort, she adds.

Dizziness

Scientists are discovering that the topsy-turvy sensations astronauts endure following prolonged space flights are similar to the dizzy feelings that many Americans experience as they age, says William H. Paloski, Ph.D., director of NASA's life sciences research laboratories at the Johnson Space Center in Houston.

For astronauts, the answer is simple—the body's balance system needs gravity to work properly. On Earth, fatigue, stress, anemia, anxiety, inner-ear infections, and other common ailments can cause dizziness. But many chronic conditions associated with aging, such as diabetes, heart disease, high blood pressure, and arteriosclerosis (hardening of the arteries), also can affect your balance, says Brian W. Blakley, M.D., chief of otolaryngology at the University of Manitoba Faculty of Medicine in Winnipeg and author of *Feeling Dizzy*. Here are a few ways to stop this topsy-turvy sensation.

Get down. For mild dizziness, the best thing you can do is lie down, relax, and wait for the dizziness to go away, Dr. Blakley suggests. Often, the sensation will disappear within a few minutes. Even if you're at some social occasion, excuse yourself, take a break, and lie down on a couch or stretch out in a lounge chair with your feet as high as possible, at least higher than your heart. You want to elevate your legs to stimulate blood flow to your brain. If there's no place to lie down, just retire for a minute—even go to the john if you have to—sit down, and lower your head between your legs until the dizziness subsides, he suggests.

Eat three squares a day. Skipping meals can result in low blood sugar, a common cause of dizziness, Dr. Blakley explains. Similarly, eating unusual fare like an all-liquid diet can create a mineral imbalance in your body that could cause wooziness. Eat at least three well-balanced meals a day consisting of 3 to 5 servings of fruits and vegetables; 6 to 11 servings of breads, cereal, and other foods made with grains; 2 to 3 servings of dairy products like milk and cheese; and 2 to 3 servings of meat and fish.

Shake the salt habit. Too much salt in the diet causes the body to retain fluid, which can disrupt the workings of the inner ear, according to Dr. Blakley. Avoid cheese, bacon, and salty snacks. Read package labels carefully and reach for foods that are advertised as having no salt added or being low in sodium or reduced sodium. Use herbs, spices, and fruit juices to season foods, he says. And be sure to rinse canned foods like tuna to remove salty juices.

Move like a snail. Rapid changes in head positions, particularly when you shift from lying down to standing up, can cause dizziness, Dr. Blakley explains. Move in stages. If you're getting out of bed, for instance, sit on the edge of the mattress for at least 30 seconds before standing.

Jump into the deep end. Practicing the very movements that cause dizziness can help your brain learn to compensate for the problem. As a starting point, Dr. Blakley suggests doing three repetitions of the following exercises,

When to See a Doctor

- Your dizziness is unexplained, severe, recurrent, or persistent.
- You also have difficulty speaking or swallowing.
- You also develop sudden weakness, numbness, or tingling on one side of your body.
- You also have a severe headache.
- Your vision suddenly gets worse or you develop double vision.
- You also have ringing in your ears or sudden loss of hearing in one ear.
- You feel dizzy after a fall or after a head injury.

three or four times a day. These exercises are designed to stimulate the balance sensors in your inner ear. They are supposed to make you dizzy and should be done while sitting in a chair or other safe place so that you will not fall if you become dizzy. Keep your eyes open.

First, try some horizontal head rotations.

1. Start in a sitting position looking straight ahead.
2. Turn your head all the way to the right, keeping your chin parallel to the floor and moving it toward your right shoulder. Then turn all the way to the left, going back and forth, slowly increasing the speed of rotation of your head as much as you can in 20 seconds.
3. Rest a few seconds.

You can also try some vertical head rotations.

1. Start in the sitting position with your head turned a little, as if you are looking at an object to your right, and your chin parallel to the floor.

2. Move your head so that your left ear moves toward your left knee. Your ear will not touch your knee in this exercise. You will have to bend your neck. Move in this direction until your head is horizontal, usually about a foot above your knee.
3. Alternate between these two positions as quickly as you can for 20 seconds.
4. Rest a few seconds.
5. Do steps 1 and 2 in the opposite direction, turning your head to the left and then moving your right ear toward your right knee. Alternate between these positions as quickly as you can for 20 seconds.

Earache

Sometimes, an earache isn't really coming from the ear. Often, ear pain is referred pain, meaning that it is really coming from somewhere else nearby. It could be a throat problem or pain from a nearby joint (the jaw, for example). Ear pain could even signal a toothache, says Charles P. Kimmelman, M.D., associate professor of otolaryngology at Weill Medical College of Cornell University in New York City and attending physician at Manhattan Eye, Ear, and Throat Hospital.

Ear pain, of course, may also mean that your ear just hurts. Sometimes, this is the result of an ear infection. To be sure of what's causing the discomfort, you should see your doctor any time you have an earache that lasts more than a day or two.

But until you get to the doctor's office, you can soothe earache pain in a number of ways.

Crank up the heat. You can use heat to treat earaches, says Michael Wynne, Ph.D., associate professor in the department of otolaryngology at the Indiana University School of Medicine in Indianapolis. Lay a warm, damp washcloth, heating pad, or hot-water bottle wrapped in a towel over the outside of your ear. You can apply the heat steadily for as long as the pain lasts. The heat over your ear will help stimulate circulation and relieve the pressure that causes the pain of earaches, Dr. Wynne says.

Drop in some oil. Put a couple of drops of warm baby oil or mineral oil in your ear canal (as long as you're certain that you've never had a ruptured eardrum), says Jennifer Derebery, M.D., otologist at the House Ear Clinic and Institute and assistant clinical professor of otolaryngology at the University of Southern California School of Medicine in Los Angeles. Once again, the warmth should soothe your pain. You can warm the oil by holding the bottle under hot water for a minute or two. Before you put the oil in your ear, put a dab on the back of your hand. If it's too hot for your hand, you can bet that it's too hot for your ear canal. After inserting the drops, wipe any excess oil off the outside of your ear.

Massage a little. Earache pain can be very sharp, so people tend to tense up, Dr. Wynne says. Relax that tension with a little light massage. Using your fingertips, apply gentle pressure and rub your jaw and neck with circular strokes for 5 to 10 minutes. Massaging the large muscle groups in the jaw and the back of the neck helps reduce tension and improves overall relaxation, thereby decreasing some of the discomfort, he says.

Quit abusing cotton swabs. Cotton-tipped swabs are fine for cleaning your outer ears, but when you start using them to clean out wax from inside your ear canal, you may as well be sending out an engraved invitation to an ear infection. So don't. Not only can swabs break the inner ear's delicate skin and make way for infection, Dr. Wynne says, they also can cause problems when they accidentally get shoved in too far or break off and damage an eardrum. And earwax, believe it or not, is a first line of defense against infection and, therefore, ear pain. Too much aggressive earwax removal clears the way for bacteria to proceed unhindered to your inner ear.

Swim smart. Getting lots of water in your ear can happen when you do a lot of swimming. That can also have an effect on your earwax, softening it, lowering its acidity, and causing the general irritation known as swimmer's ear. To combat this problem, you can use earplugs while swimming.

Some people are prone to swimmer's ear and can even get it from showering. Putting a few drops of the product Swim Ear or rubbing alcohol in your ear canal can dry up the moisture that leads to swimmer's ear. Better yet, mix a solution that is 50 percent alcohol and 50 percent white vinegar. Use an eyedropper to put a couple of drops of the solution in your ear after swimming, Dr. Wynne suggests. The alcohol helps evaporate the water that can lead to irritation, and the vinegar helps keep the acidic value of the ear canal high.

Clear your tubes. If you have a cold or flu and have to be flying, think about taking a decongestant a half-hour before you board (and before you land, if your flight will last longer than the effect of the medication) to help keep the eustachian tubes in your ears clear,

When to See a Doctor

- You have ear pain after any kind of blow to the ear.
- Your ear pain is accompanied by dizziness, loss of hearing on one side, headaches, and facial paralysis.

suggests Dr. Wynne. It is the blockage in these tubes, which lead from your ear to your nose, that make it difficult for your ears to adjust to altitude changes. That allows pressure to build up behind your eardrums, causing pain.

Keep your jaw flapping. Any time you face a change in altitude and pressure, do things that keep you swallowing, says Dr. Wynne. That opens the eustachian tubes and thus can prevent ear pain. Chew gum, yawn, sip a drink—it all helps equalize the pressure that builds in your ears when the plane is ascending or descending.

Eye, Burning

Tearing just might be one of the biggest tricks that your eyes can play on you. That's because one common cause of a watery eye is a dry eye.

Huh? That's what Robert Abel Jr., M.D., clinical professor of ophthalmology at Thomas Jefferson University in Philadelphia, says: Tearing often is brought on by dry eyes.

The liquid in the eyes comes in different forms. There are the gushy tears that spill down your face when you chop onions. These come from the lacrimal glands and are almost always in abundant supply. Then there are the tears that lubricate your eyeballs. They come from the accessory lacrimal gland. If there aren't enough tears in the accessory lacrimal gland, small dry spots form on the eyes. This irritation causes the main lacrimal gland to be stimulated, leaving you with watery eyes, according to Dr. Abel.

Another cause of watery eyes is allergies. The immune system triggers the release of histamine, which is a chemical that causes the eyes to tear, itch, and get bloodshot. Chemicals such as fiberglass and the chlorine in swimming pools can cause similar reactions.

Before you can dry watery eyes, you have to know what's making them water in the first place. If it's allergies, you'll probably have other symptoms, like sneezing or a stuffy nose. If you suspect dry eyes, ask your ophthalmologist to perform a filter paper test. A piece of filter paper is placed on the eye for 5 minutes. Then the doctor measures how many tears your eye produced.

Whatever's causing your dry eyes, here are a few tips that can help.

Go fish. Dietary substances such as glucosamine sulfate, essential fatty acids, and B vitamins will help keep your whole body, including the eyes, moist and lubricated. You can get these nutrients by eating more cold-water fish or using flaxseed oil. Or you can take supplements. "I take essential fatty acids once or twice a day. What I have found is that my skin is more moist. My eyes don't seem dry. And in the winter, I don't get a dry cough," says Dr. Abel.

Don't rub. "For 5 seconds, it feels really good. And then it burns like hell," says Dr. Abel. The burning sensation that you experience comes from oil on your eyelid. When you rub the other side of the lid, you turn the oil into a thick, viscous tear film that burns.

Take a break. People who work at computers tend to get dry eyes. "When you do a lot of close work, you tend to stare. That dries out your eyes and makes them uncomfortable," says Dr. Abel.

Take an eye break every 20 minutes, advises James L. Cox, a behavioral optometrist in Bellflower, California. Look away from what you are doing and focus on something at least 15 feet away—across the room, down the hallway, out the window—to give your eyes a chance to rest.

Fatigue

Fatigue is one of the most common reasons that we consult our family doctors. And that's not surprising when you consider the number of conditions that have fatigue as a symptom. Stress, depression, thyroid problems, anemia, and food allergies can all cause persistent tiredness, says Susan M. Lark, M.D., author of *Chronic Fatigue and Tiredness* and director of the PMS and Menopause Self-Help Center in Los Altos, California. Many women also have premenstrual fatigue or fatigue that's related to menopause. And while it may seem obvious, many of us simply don't get enough sleep.

If your fatigue continues for 6 months or longer and is so severe that you can't function normally, you may have chronic fatigue syndrome, a mysterious illness that causes flu-like symptoms, persistent muscle pain, and problems remembering or concentrating. It hits mostly people between ages 25 and 50 and is relatively rare. Experts estimate that only 1 in 30 fatigued people has chronic fatigue syndrome.

There are a number of vitamins and minerals that play roles in keeping you fatigue-free. Try these.

Reach for iron. One of the most common causes of fatigue for women is iron-deficiency anemia, says Dr. Lark. She estimates that 20 percent of women who menstruate are anemic because of the blood they lose each month. "Women with heavy menstrual flow have the greatest risk," she adds. Anemia is also common among teenagers, pregnant women, and women nearing menopause. Make an appointment with your doctor to find out for sure.

But even if you're not anemic, a slight iron deficiency can affect your energy level, says Dr. Lark. Experts generally suggest between 12 and 15 milligrams a day. The best source of iron is animal products, so go for lean meats and cooked oysters and clams. Some vegetables such as spinach, as well as legumes such as green beans, lima beans, and pinto beans are also rich in iron, but the type found in them is not as easy to absorb as that from animal sources.

If you're a vegetarian, drinking some orange juice or taking a vitamin C supplement of at least 75 milligrams along with iron-rich vegetables will help your body absorb more iron from your food, says Dr. Lark. Many commercial breads and breakfast cereals are also fortified with iron.

Turn to a dynamic duo. Potassium and magnesium are two minerals that may be beneficial for persistent fatigue, says Dr. Lark. She recommends trying between 100 and 200 milligrams of each mineral for up to 6 months to see if they alleviate fatigue. It's safe for anyone in good health, she says, although people with heart or kidney problems or diabetes shouldn't take these minerals without consulting a doctor first.

Rev up with vitamin C. Some studies suggest low vitamin C intake can also contribute to fatigue. Dr. Lark recommends about 4,000 milligrams of vitamin C a day for people with persistent fatigue. She warns that this high dose can cause temporary diarrhea in some people. "If this happens," she says, "just cut back on the dose to the point where the diarrhea goes away."

Stay on the wagon. "Alcohol is a central nervous system depressant, which is the last thing you need if you are feeling chronically tired," says Dr. Lark.

Don't lean on caffeine. It's tempting to reach for a cup of strong coffee, but it's likely to give you a temporary jolt of energy and then let you down. Instead, Dr. Lark recommends a caffeine-free herbal tea containing ginger root. "It tastes good and is mildly stimulating, but there's no rebound effect," she says.

Master your sugar cravings. Simple sugars, such as those found in cookies, candies, and desserts, cause sharp increases in your blood sugar level, which may make you feel temporarily energized. But after the initial rush, blood sugar drops sharply, says Dr. Lark, which can result in an energy crisis.

Lighten up on fat. "Fatty foods, including most meats, are very hard to digest," says Dr. Lark. She recommends a low-fat diet high in whole grains, legumes, and fresh fruits and vegetables.

Foot Odor

Right now, as you read this, millions of microscopic creatures are living on your feet. It might give you the heebie-jeebies to think about it, but these bacteria are perfectly normal inhabitants for feet to have. In fact, they know something that never occurred to you: Your feet are a great feasting ground. But if you overfeed them, they can really start to stink up the place.

"With sweating and high temperatures, your skin will flake. Bacteria will feed on these flakes," says Walter J. Pedowitz, M.D., associate clinical professor of orthopedic surgery at Columbia University in New York City. That would be fine if they cleaned up after themselves. But instead, the feasting bacteria produce organic substances called fatty acids, and those are the leftovers that start to reek on your feet.

Thankfully, the aging process gives you some natural protection against foot odor. You have 3,000 sweat glands per square inch of skin on your feet. Over the years, these sweat glands release less and less sweat. Less sweat means less food for bacteria. So teenagers and young adults usually have more problems with foot odor than people who are 60-plus.

Foot odor may also signal an infection. People with diabetes often have dry, cracked skin on their feet. These cracks provide footholds for yeast, bacteria, and fungi to set up camp. Left uncontrolled, these cases of athlete's foot and other skin infections can smell. At that point, you may need to see your doctor, who can prescribe an antifungal ointment.

But for everyday smell protection, there are ways to keep those little inhabitants in check and keep your feet smelling fresh.

Throw out those stinking shoes. No matter what you do to make your feet smell better, if you shove them back inside a pair of smelly shoes, they'll stink all over again. So get rid of them and treat yourself to a new pair, says Dr. Pedowitz.

Change shoes and socks often. Aim to change your shoes and socks at least once a day. But gauge your shoe and sock changes by how much your feet sweat. As soon as you notice that they are wet, it's time for a change. Wash each pair of socks after wearing them. Try to rotate your shoes so they have a day to dry out between wearings, advises Dr. Pedowitz.

Buy absorbent socks. Thick, soft socks will soak up the sweat, keeping it away from your skin. Stay away from nylon, which doesn't breathe or absorb moisture but does pick up odor fast, says Dr. Pedowitz.

Add inserts. Sold over the counter, shoe inserts such as Odor-Eaters are widely available and can help keep your feet odor-free, notes Dr. Pedowitz.

Apply some powder. Dust your feet with baby or foot powder. The powder will absorb some of the sweat, adds Dr. Pedowitz.

Buy breathable shoes. A leather shoe isn't the best thing you can put on your foot. Once odor gets into leather shoes, it won't get out. They're ruined. Plus, leather makes your feet sweat. So opt for canvas or nylon shoes that have as little leather as possible, says Alan J. Liftin, M.D., a dermatologist in private practice in Livingston, New Jersey.

Wash what you can. In addition to washing your socks, also remember to take out any inserts or pads in your shoes and wash those regularly too, Dr. Liftin says.

Take a tea bath. If your problem is excess sweating, soak your feet in a bucket of strongly brewed black tea, says Dr. Pedowitz. The tannic acid in the tea will kill the bacteria and close down your pores, keeping your feet dry longer. Use two tea bags per pint of water and boil for 15 minutes. Then remove the bags and add 2 quarts of water to the tea. Soak your feet for 30 minutes daily for about a week.

Foot Pain

When your feet have a problem, they'll let you know it. First, they send you signals like calluses, black toenails, and bunions. If you deal only with the signals or the symptoms but don't solve the underlying problem, your feet will eventually send you another message that's impossible to overlook: pain.

Usually, the problem in question is that your shoes don't fit right or that you were born with certain foot problems that need to be corrected by a doctor, says Neil Scheffler, D.P.M., podiatrist and president of health care and education for the Mid-Atlantic Region of the American Association of Diabetes in Baltimore. Other factors, however, also come into play. For instance, putting on extra weight as you age can add a tremendous amount of pressure to your feet.

Regardless of why your feet hurt, here are some strategies to nip pain in the bud.

Stomp on pain. Nonsteroidal anti-inflammatory drugs such as ibuprofen can relieve the pain and swelling of most types of foot pain. Follow package directions. This is a temporary fix, however. You don't want to stay on over-the-counter painkillers for more than a few weeks, advises Tzvi Bar-David, D.P.M., a podiatrist with Columbia-Presbyterian Medical Center in New York City. So make sure to try other strategies to relieve your specific foot problem.

Bend some toes to stretch a tendon. If your pain stems from a tight Achilles tendon, stretching it can help. Get in a relaxed position—sitting or lying down—and bend your leg until your toes are within reach. Using both hands, pull your toes toward your shin and hold for 20 seconds.

Or lean in for tendon relief. Another Achilles tendon stretch can be done standing up in front of a wall. Place your hands against the wall and lean forward with your feet firmly planted flat on the ground behind you. Keep your back and feet flat and your knees locked. You will feel your calf stretching if you do this properly, notes Dr. Bar-David. Repeat this 10 times, holding each stretch for 30 seconds.

Vary your stretch times. The Achilles tendon stretches can help alleviate heel pain when it strikes, but you should also do them routinely. Be sure to stretch before and after exercising. Also, stretch before going to sleep and before getting out of bed in the morning. Though you might think your legs and feet are relaxed at night, most people sleep with their feet pointed, keeping the muscles tight all night long, Dr. Bar-David says. By stretching before you rise, you can get your feet off to a good start.

Cushion that heel. Shop around for heel cups or ask a podiatrist about some cushioning that will make your heel feel better. With extra cushioning, your heels aren't jarred so much by everyday walking or running. And with the slight heel lift, your Achilles tendon has a chance to relax, explains Dr. Bar-David.

Switch to running or walking shoes. If your foot's natural padding has eroded over time, wear sneakers. They have extra cushioning in the heel, which helps make up for your somewhat reduced, natural fat pads, says James Michelson, M.D., associate professor of orthopedic surgery at Johns Hopkins School of Medicine in Baltimore. Lace-up shoes also will put less stress on the front of your foot if you have pain there.

Lose weight. If you've gained weight over the years, common sense tells you the extra pounds are putting extra pressure on your feet. This can create heel or forefoot pain, warns Dr. Bar-David. The lighter your body, the less your foot pain.

Get cushioned inserts. You can buy inserts to put in the sole of your shoe to absorb more shock. "Usually, it's all that's needed," adds Dr. Michelson.

Go for depth. If inserts and running shoes don't do the trick, go to a specialty orthopedic shoe store and ask for shoes that provide extra depth. These will allow you to stick even more cushioned inserts into your shoe to absorb even more shock, according to Dr. Michelson.

Avoid high heels. For women, wearing high heels could contribute to arthritis and other foot pain. High heels also push all of the force of walking into the front of your foot, where things are tight and immovable. Switch to flats, says Dr. Michelson.

Get your feet measured. Shoes that are too tight will make your feet hurt even more. Most women wear their shoes two sizes too small, notes Dr. Michelson, and many haven't had their feet measured in at least 5 years. Since your feet grow as you age, the shoe that fit when you were 40 may be too small now. Have a clerk or a friend measure your feet for you while you are standing. And do this every time you buy a new pair of shoes, advises Dr. Michelson.

Shop at the end of the day. Your feet swell over the course of the day and you'll want shoes that fit when your feet are at their largest.

Keep in mind that one foot might be larger than the other. When you're shoe shopping, always fit shoes to your larger foot. (Use cushioning, if necessary, to fill in the gaps in the shoe for your smaller foot.) Make sure there's at least a half-inch between your longest toe and the end of the shoe.

Make ginger a habit. Fresh ginger is a great remedy for arthritis and other pain related to swelling, because it's a natural anti-inflammatory, says Neal Barnard, M.D., author of *Foods That Fight Pain* and president of the Physicians Committee for Responsible Medicine in Washington, D.C. Though you don't have to use a lot of it to get significant relief, you do have to take it regularly, he says.

Buy fresh ginger at the supermarket. Mince up ½ to 1 teaspoon per day. Either put it in your food as a flavoring or mix it into some water and swallow it like a pill. Cloves, garlic, and turmeric, though less studied, have shown similar effects in some people, according to Dr. Barnard.

Rub hot peppers on them. Over-the-counter creams made from capsaicin, the active ingredient in hot peppers, can relieve arthritis and other foot pain, says Dr. Barnard. The lotion may at first cause a burning sensation, which goes away the more you use the stuff. Rub just enough to lightly cover the affected area on your feet whenever you feel pain. Wash your hands thoroughly after each application and keep the cream away from your eyes and other mucous membranes. It can really burn.

Modify your exercise. If your feet hurt because you give them a regular pounding every time you take a brisk walk, change your routine, says Donna Astion, M.D., associate chief of foot and ankle service for the Hospital for Joint Diseases, Orthopaedic Institute in New York City. For instance, try taking every other day off, alternating between weight-bearing activities such as running and nonweight-bearing activities such as cycling. If you run, alternate between hard tar roads and softer surfaces like trails.

Soak them. Treat your feet to a soak in Epsom salts and warm water. The soak can drain swollen tissues and help relieve pressure. Follow the directions on the package, which usually recommend 1 tablespoon of Epsom salts dissolved in each quart of water.

Forgetfulness

Within your brain are hundreds of billions of cells called neurons that stretch toward each other with rootlike growths called axons and dendrites. Close as they might get, the tiny nerve endings of one axon never touch those of the dendrites branching toward it. Instead, memories and other thoughts have to hurdle what are called synaptic gaps.

Without chemicals called neurotransmitters (such as dopamine, norepinephrine, serotonin, and acetylcholine) bridging these gaps, information just can't get from one neuron to the other. And that means memories, though stored throughout your brain, are just out of reach. Although the brain's primary fuel is glucose, experts believe that key vitamins and minerals supply the raw material for many of these neurotransmitters. Here's how to up your intake of them.

Benefit from B$_6$. Vitamin B$_6$ (also called pyridoxine) apparently helps create important neurotransmitters, says Michael Ebadi, Ph.D., professor of pharmacology and neurology at the University of Nebraska College of Medicine in Omaha.

The Daily Value of 2 milligrams should be sufficient to help keep your memory in good working order. You can easily get this amount as part of a B-complex supplement. You should never take B_6 by itself without medical supervision, as amounts above 100 milligrams can be toxic.

Boost the brain with B_{12}. "B_{12} deficiency causes problems in the nervous system, including burning points in the feet and mental problems such as difficulty with recent memory and the ability to calculate," says Sally Stabler, M.D., associate professor of medicine at the University of Colorado Health Sciences Center School of Medicine in Denver. A B_{12} deficiency has even been known to change brain wave activity, she says.

Nearly one-third of people over 60 can't extract the vitamin B_{12} they need from what they eat. That's because their stomachs no longer secrete enough gastric acid, which breaks down food and helps turn it into fuel for your brain and body.

And taking supplements won't help, because they are also broken down in the stomach. So doctors who suspect vitamin B_{12} deficiencies in people with memory problems give them B_{12} shots, thus bypassing the faltering digestive system.

Vitamin B_{12} deficiency caused by diet is rare when the digestive system is in good working order. That's because eating just small portions of dairy products or animal protein gives you enough of this vital nutrient. About the only eating plan that seems to put you at risk are diets that completely eliminate meats and dairy products. But even then you have to adhere to such a diet for at least several years before a deficiency develops, says Dr. Stabler.

Virtually all animal products, such as milk, cheeses, yogurt, and lean beef contain vitamin B_{12}. The Daily Value for B_{12} is 6 micrograms.

Try fortification at its finest. Both thiamin and riboflavin, other important B vitamins, are routinely added to most flours, cereals, and grain products. Even mild deficiencies of these vitamins can have an impact on your thinking and memory.

Fortunately, it doesn't take much thiamin to make a difference. One study showed that women who were restricted to 0.33 milligram of thiamin a day became irritable, fatigued, and unsociable. These symptoms improved with just 1.4 milligrams of thiamin a day. The Daily Value for thiamin is 1.5 milligrams, while the Daily Value for riboflavin is 1.7 milligrams.

Make the lecithin-choline connection. Lecithin is a common food additive used in ice cream, margarine, mayonnaise, and chocolate bars to help wed the fat in these foods with water. It has healthful qualities as well, such as mildly increasing the amount of choline in your brain. And more choline means more acetylcholine, an important neurotransmitter that you need for your memory to function.

"The fascinating thing about lecithin is that when it helps, it's right away," says Florence Safford, Ph.D., professor of social work and gerontology at Florida International University in Miami. Dr. Safford recommends 2 tablespoons of lecithin granules a day. Just mix it in with foods such as yogurt, applesauce, and cereals.

Think with iron and zinc. While researchers have established the importance of iron and zinc in the mental development of infants, you have to dig into the scientific literature before you'll find studies showing that these minerals help make for better memories in adults as well. In one small preliminary study, women who took iron supplements had better short-term verbal memory, while visual memory, or the ability to remember pictures, was improved by both zinc and iron.

Keep the Memories Flowing

It's easy with these dietary tips.

Control your cocktails. Excessive drinking can deplete your body's stores of B vitamins, says Michael Ebadi, Ph.D., professor of pharmacology and neurology at the University of Nebraska College of Medicine in Omaha. "There is a whole syndrome of B vitamin and zinc deficiencies that occurs in alcoholics, causing memory loss and even seizures," he says.

Also, drinking often takes the place of healthy eating, thus lowering the amounts of essential nutrients that you eat. Alcohol can also make it difficult for the body to digest and absorb nutrients. Make sure that you don't have more than two drinks a day, says Dr. Ebadi.

Eat low-fat. Details from the famous Framingham Heart Study show that the higher the blood pressure, the lower the scores on a series of mental tests, including memory tests. Researchers theorize that higher blood pressure may cause changes in blood flow to the brain. One proven strategy to bring down high blood pressure is to eat a diet that gets no more than 25 percent of its calories from fat.

Although the women received supplements during the study, foods are much better sources of these nutrients, says Harold Sandstead, M.D., professor in the department of preventive medicine and community health at the University of Texas Medical Branch at Galveston. Steamed clams, Cream of Wheat cereal, and soybeans are all good sources of iron, while whole grains, wheat bran, wheat germ, meats, and oysters and other seafood are top sources of zinc. For a double punch, try pumpkin seeds. They're high sources of both iron and zinc.

Women who menstruate need between 2 and 2.5 milligrams of iron a day to offset loss of the mineral, explains Dr. Sandstead. (The Daily Value for iron is much higher—18 milligrams—because your body doesn't absorb all of the mineral that you take in.) "If they have heavy menstrual loss, the level goes up even more," he adds. Men need about 1 milligram of iron a day. Experts believe that pumping up your iron intake helps build those all-important brain neurotransmitters, among other things.

And how does zinc help memory? Apparently, vitamin B_6 can't do its job without zinc pitching in, says Dr. Ebadi. "In the absence of zinc, active B_6 is not formed properly in the brain, and as a result, neither are key neurotransmitters," he says. Not only that, but large amounts of zinc have been found in the brain's memory center, the hippocampus. The Daily Value for zinc is 15 milligrams.

Gas

It's embarrassing, to be sure, but don't necessarily view gas as a health problem, says Roger L. Gebhard, M.D., gastroenterologist at the Veterans Affairs Medical Center and professor of medicine in the division of gastroenterology at the University of Minnesota, both in Minneapolis. Most of us produce roughly 1 to 3 pints of gas daily, and the only way to relieve that pressure is through burping or flatulence. "The average person passes gas 14 to 20 times a day," Dr. Gebhard says, "which may seem like a lot, but it's actually perfectly normal."

Still, you'd probably prefer to decrease the likelihood of embarrassing episodes. There are a number of simple things you can do to ward off rumblings from down under, says Dr. Gebhard. If flatulence keeps you grumbling, here's how to keep it under control.

Ration the gas supply. "Most flatulence originates in the carbohydrates of foods we eat," says Dr. Gebhard. "If there are certain foods that you suspect are causing the flatulence, cut those foods out of your diet for 3 days to see if it reduces the problem. By that time, you'll know, and you can quickly use trial and error to discover the worst offenders."

Here's what's going on. Remember that 1 to 3 pints of gas we mentioned? Most of it is produced by harmless bacteria living in your large intestine, Dr. Gebhard says. Whenever you eat a carbohydrate, your digestive system can't fully break it down. The bacteria living there will do it for you, but this produces gas as a by-product.

Depending on which particular carbohydrates you eat or enzymes you may lack (most often the lactase that breaks down dairy products), a number of different foods could cause problems with flatulence. Beans, vegetables high in cellulose (like broccoli and cauliflower), dairy products, and foods or supplements high in fiber are the most common problems, says Dr. Gebhard. Of course, all these contribute to a healthy diet, he points out, so you don't want to eliminate them completely. But cutting back on the one causing the most problems may make a big difference.

Stop milking it for all it's worth. You may have discovered that milk as well as milk products like cheese and ice cream seem to trigger a lot of gas. That's understandable. As we grow older, our bodies produce less of an enzyme called lactase that breaks down the natural sugar in milk called lactose. Lack of that enzyme also causes gas.

If you still like milk for a good dose of bone-strengthening calcium, take it with an over-the-counter lactose digestion aid such as Lactaid, says Harris Clearfield, M.D., professor of medicine and director of the division of gastroenterology at Hahnemann University Hospital in Philadelphia. They help your body digest the lactose before any bacteria can get to it. Also, most supermarkets offer reduced-lactose milk or cheese.

Break down the beans. You can turn down the volume of certain hard-to-digest beans by adding a few drops of Beano to your food, says Dr. Gebhard. Beano works to break down the complex sugar found in those foods, making life simpler for your digestive system. Look for it in supermarkets and drug stores.

Give them a good soak. Another way to stifle those problematic beans is to soak them in a pot of water overnight, then pour out the water and refill the pot before cooking, says James Duke, Ph.D., botanical consultant, author of *The Green Pharmacy*, and a former ethnobotanist with the U.S. Department of Agriculture who specializes in medicinal plants. This helps to remove the offending carbohydrates. Better yet, add a small whole carrot to the pot of beans after soaking them, he suggests. Carrots can help soothe the digestive tract.

Swallow smartly. The amount of air that you swallow can have a big impact on how much gas you pass, although most of it will come out as belches, says Dr. Gebhard. When you eat and drink rapidly, you tend to swallow air without realizing it, he says. You also gulp down too much air when you chew gum, suck on hard candy, or smoke. And some people gulp air just because they're nervous, so that's another thing to watch out for. Also, ill-fitting dentures can lead to higher amounts of air-swallowing. So if you wear dentures, it might be worth checking with a dentist to make sure they fit properly.

Meanwhile, slow down when you're having dinner, sip rather than gulp, and try to be aware of times when you tend to swallow air, Dr. Gebhard suggests. As a last resort, become one of those people who constantly chews on a pen. The pen will keep your teeth separated, making it virtually impossible to swallow large amounts of air.

Say good-bye to soda. The carbonation in soft drinks, seltzer water, beer, and other carbonated beverages can cause gas problems, says Dr. Clearfield. It's gas that keeps the beverages bubbly, and when that gas goes to your inner gut, it still has the fizz in it. Stay away from these beverages for a few days to see if your symptoms improve, he suggests.

Stick with it. Any new addition to your diet like a high-fiber supplement or eight-bean chili recipe may cause flatulence in the short term. But if you continue to get your fill of fiber, your body may adjust, says Dr. Gebhard. So if a food or supplement is important to your health, don't give it up because of a one-time gas attack. Start small and gradually increase the amount you're taking in, he recommends. You might try adding about 5 grams of fiber more than you're used to each day for 1 week, then an additional 5 the next week, and so on until you are consuming 25 to 35 grams of fiber per day. Over time, your body might produce less gas in response.

Stamp out sorbitol. Sorbitol, another sugar that our bodies have trouble digesting, is used as an artificial sweetener in sugar-free gums, candies, and many dietetic foods, reports Dr. Gebhard. It's also found naturally in certain fruits such as apples, pears, prunes, and peaches, but only the concentrated form packed into food products causes flatulence problems. If you consume a lot of these products, try cutting back, he suggests.

Spice things up. Herbs known as carminatives may help the problem by soothing the digestive tract, says Dr. Duke. Among these are anise seed, basil, bergamot, coriander, dill, fennel, lemon balm, marjoram, oregano, peppermint, rosemary, sage, and thyme. Adding a touch of one or more of these herbs to your food or tea can be a flavorful way to solve the problem.

Choose charcoal. Activated charcoal tablets are an over-the-counter solution that may absorb gas and provide some relief, says Dr. Clearfield. While the medical evidence for charcoal's effectiveness is still somewhat murky, there's no harm in giving it a try, he says. Follow the package directions for dosage. Just don't be alarmed if your stools turn black. It's a common result of taking the tablets.

Genital Irritation

An estimated 75 percent of women get at least one yeast infection during their lives. To deal with yeast infection, many women head for the local drugstore and buy an over-the-counter treatment such as miconazole nitrate (Monistat). But if treatments address only vaginal symptoms, you're getting at only half of the problem, says Lorilee Schoenbeck, N.D., a naturopathic doctor with the Champlain Centers for Natural Medicine in Shelburne and Middlebury, Vermont.

When it comes to chronic or recurring infections, the heart of the problem is often the intestines rather than the vaginal area, according to many naturopaths. *Candida albicans*, the organism that most frequently causes yeast infections, can sometimes become overgrown in your intestines. Yeast that exits the gastrointestinal tract can migrate into the vagina. That area can become infected repeatedly, says Dr. Schoenbeck.

Yeast infections can also mimic urinary tract infections or sexually transmitted diseases, so it's important to get an accurate diagnosis from a medical practitioner before beginning treatment. Also, you should definitely consult your doctor if this is your first experience with symptoms of a yeast infection or if you are pregnant and have an underlying condition such as diabetes. Your doctor can determine whether you have a yeast infection.

Fortunately, there are many things that you can do to ward off yeast infections in the first place.

Limit your sweets. Candida breeds even more profusely when you ingest a lot of sugar, says Dr. Schoenbeck.

Spell d-r-y. Candida loves a warm, moist environment. Panty hose, tight jeans, wet bathing suits, and sweaty exercise clothes all provide the yeast with an ideal set of moist conditions. If you get damp clothes off as fast as you can and change into something dry and airy, you just might discourage the little diehards. Also, wear only pure cotton underwear, says Dr. Schoenbeck.

Get the right stuff: acidophilus. Because the vaginal itching, redness, and pain can drive you absolutely nuts, you have to take care of the immediate outbreak first, says Dr. Schoenbeck. *Lactobacillus acidophilus* is your ally because it's a type of good bacteria that helps keep candida in check.

When the level of acidophilus is down, candida starts growing like wild. This is frequently the case if you have recently taken antibiotics for an infection or are continuously taking them for acne. In the process of killing off infectious bacteria, antibiotics inadvertently kill off acidophilus as well. One way to get more acidophilus is to eat live-culture yogurt. Acidophilus also comes in supplement form.

Acidophilus capsules can help re-establish normal intestinal health, says Dr. Schoenbeck. Take the capsules only when you have an active yeast infection or are having a problem with recurring infections.

Taking oral doses of acidophilus for just 2 to 4 weeks can help decrease candida in both your vagina and your intestines, she says. That makes you less prone to repeat infections.

Look for acidophilus capsules that are refrigerated and contain at least one billion organisms per capsule. Dr. Schoenbeck recommends two capsules before breakfast and two before dinner, 1 hour before each meal, for 1 month. At the end of the month, see your medical practitioner to be certain that the infection is gone.

Acidophilus capsules can also help with prevention. If your doctor prescribes antibiotics, you can help prevent a yeast outbreak by starting the acidophilus capsules at the same time as your prescription. Continue taking the capsules for just 2 weeks, says Dr. Schoenbeck.

Turn to garlic. "Garlic is one of the best things to take for yeast infections," says naturopathic doctor Tori Hudson, N.D., professor at the National College of Naturopathic Medicine in Portland, Oregon, and author of *Women's Encyclopedia of Natural Medicine*. It is both antifungal and immunity-boosting, she says.

Two garlic capsules a day are enough to protect against yeast, according to Dr. Hudson. It's best to take enteric-coated capsules because the coating prevents the active ingredients in garlic from breaking down in the stomach. Look for garlic capsules with 4,000 milligrams of allicin-alliin, which is the antifungal agent found in garlic, she says.

Reach for other herbs. Oregon grape root extract, tea tree oil extract, and lavender extract all help reduce the amount of candida growing in the intestines. "There are supplements that contain all of these extracts, but they are hard to find. I'd ask an alternative practitioner to prescribe one," Dr. Schoenbeck says. She recommends taking two tablets three times a day. After a month, see your practitioner to be sure the infection is gone.

Echinacea is beneficial, too. A German study found that women taking antifungal medicine plus echinacea extract had only a 10 percent recurrence of yeast infections. Another great anti-yeast herb is goldenseal, says Dr. Schoenbeck. It contains a chemical that has antibiotic properties and works particularly well against yeast. You can buy echinacea and goldenseal separately or in combination capsules. Whichever you choose, take them daily as directed on the product you buy. If the capsules are 450 milligrams of an echinacea and goldenseal combination, a typical dose would be two or three capsules daily with water. Do not use goldenseal if you are pregnant, however.

Drinking a tea made with pau d'arco bark or taking a supplement may also bring relief, says Kathleen Head, N.D., a naturopathic doctor in Sandpoint, Idaho, and senior editor of *Alternative Medicine Review*.

Gums, Bleeding

What if you floss and brush until you're blue in the face and you still have bleeding, receding gums?

You're dealing with a stubborn case of gingivitis. And it is cause for concern. Left for even a short time along your gum line, food particles and bacteria combine to form plaque, which hardens on your teeth and irritates your gums. Irritated gums bleed and eventually start to recede, creating pockets next to your teeth. Before long, the plaque starts attacking the roots of your teeth and your jawbone; this is the point at which gingivitis turns into a more serious gum problem known as periodontal disease. If it progresses too far without proper medical intervention, you might even lose some teeth.

In addition to regular dental visits, use these tips to keep your gums healthy.

Take C and see improvement. "Vitamin C is the one nutrient that has been shown to have quite a positive effect on the mouth when in adequate levels in the body," says Cherilyn Sheets, D.D.S., a spokesperson for the

Academy of General Dentistry and a dentist in Newport Beach, California. People with vitamin C deficiencies can have some of the worst gum and dental problems that dentists see.

Research with laboratory animals confirms that vitamin C deficiency causes gum swelling, decreased mineral content of the jawbone, and loose teeth. Why the damage? Vitamin C is vital for production of collagen, the basic protein building block for the fibrous framework of all tissues, including gums, explains Mary Dan Eades, M.D., medical director of the Arkansas Center for Health and Weight Control in Little Rock. "Vitamin C strengthens weak gum tissue and makes the gum lining more resistant to penetration by bacteria," she says.

Dr. Eades recommends using vitamin C in two ways—as a mouthwash and as a supplement—to fight gingivitis. "Mix ½ teaspoon of crystalline vitamin C with a sugar-free citrus beverage, swish the mixture in your mouth for 1 minute, then swallow, twice daily," she advises. Follow each rinse with plenty of fresh water.

Crystalline vitamin C (powdered pure ascorbic acid) is available in health food stores. Chewable or powdered vitamin C can erode tooth enamel. So it's best to stick to the crystalline form if you're using it as a mouth rinse.

You can also take 500-milligram slow-release vitamin C capsules, one or two in the morning and one or two in the evening, says Dr. Eades. (Some people may experience diarrhea when taking vitamin C in doses exceeding 1,200 milligrams a day.) Meanwhile, keep on brushing and flossing!

Phase out soft drinks. Canned soda contains excess phosphorus, a mineral that could lead to the leaching of calcium from your bones, a potential cause of osteoporosis. Some researchers believe that calcium is first robbed not from your hips or spine but from your jaw, leading to tooth loss, says Ken Wical, D.D.S., professor of restorative dentistry at Loma Linda University in California.

Reduce your sugar. In addition to promoting dental decay, sugar is thought to harm gums. Many dentists believe that sugar feeds the bacteria that cause the infection leading to gingivitis, although there are no definitive studies to prove this.

Hair Loss

Not all hair loss is inevitable, nor is the decline entirely controlled by genes. Stress, hormone changes, and vitamin or mineral deficiencies can lead to fast fallout. Moreover, you're likely to lose hair faster if your hair follicles become inflamed or if you get skin disorders that affect your scalp.

Women aren't immune to some of the fallout from these problems. "I've had women patients who have lost all their hair due to major stresses in their lives," says Hope Fay, N.D., a naturopathic doctor in Seattle. "When you're under stress from illness or work, sometimes the circulation in the scalp is so constricted that the hair follicles lose blood supply, which causes them to die and fall out." Dr. Fay is quick to add, however, that if women lose their hair, it often grows right back in when they're no longer under extreme stress.

To help the hair return when the loss isn't a matter of inherited baldness, try these tactics.

Mine minerals. Deficiencies of selenium and zinc generally lead to hair loss, researchers have observed. These minerals aid in immune function and in the utilization of protein that your body needs to help produce hair.

Normally, you get these trace minerals through plant foods. "Unfortunately, in some areas of the United States, some trace minerals just aren't in the soil in high enough quantities. You could eat what you think is a good diet but still be lacking," says Elizabeth Wotton, N.D., a naturopathic doctor at Compass Family Health Center in Plymouth, Massachusetts.

If that's your problem, pick up a trace mineral supplement. It should include a wide variety of trace minerals, including amounts such as 200 micrograms of selenium and 20 milligrams of zinc.

"Follow the dosage directions on the bottle and try it for several weeks," says Dr. Wotton. "It will be a while before you know if it's working."

You can also take 30 milligrams of zinc daily and see if you stop losing hair or even start to grow it back, says Dr. Wotton. If your hair loss is due to a zinc deficiency, you could see regrowth in as little as a week. Talk to a doctor before taking this amount of zinc, however.

Pluck nettle. This herb is really high in mineral content and can make your hair much healthier, Dr. Fay says.

Nettle comes in a tincture or capsules. In either form, simply follow the dosage directions on the bottle. For 480-milligram capsules, for example, the typical dose is one capsule twice a day. A typical tincture dose is 15 to 20 drops in ¼ cup of water or juice twice a day.

Regulate hormones. In the first few months after their children are born, some women find that their hair begins to fall out. The problem is usually due to hormonal changes. The body's hormone ratios are radically revised during pregnancy. After delivery, the body has to establish a new balance.

Hormone upsets aren't limited to new mothers, however. Stress, menopause, and illness can also bring on changes.

To ease hormonal transitions, Dr. Wotton suggests eating more foods containing phytoestrogens, plant compounds that mimic the biological activities of female hormones. These foods include legumes and soy products, such as tofu.

Dr. Wotton also suggests supplementing your diet with a few important minerals and vitamins. She recommends 150 milligrams of magnesium twice a day, 400 to 800 international units of vitamin E daily, and a daily vitamin B-complex supplement that contains 100 milligrams of B_6 and 50 micrograms of biotin.

"With these supplements, you're giving your body all the right raw materials," Dr. Wotton says. "If hormones are your problem, your body should eventually right itself."

Supplement with fatty acids. Essential fatty acids from flaxseed oil or evening primrose oil form the biological backbone of many hormone molecules, says Dr. Fay. The oils are rich sources of omega-3 and omega-6 fatty acids, good fats that are important for healthy skin and hair.

Dr. Fay suggests taking 1,000 milligrams of evening primrose oil three times a day or 1 teaspoon of flaxseed oil once or twice a day. You can take the flaxseed oil by the spoonful or put it on salads and other foods.

Headache

More than 90 percent of all headaches are classified as tension headaches, which occur when the muscles in the back of your neck and scalp tighten. When you have a tension headache, you feel a generalized dull head pain. That's a signal that the nerves running through the muscles have become inflamed and irritated.

Migraines are another kind of animal. The pulsating throb of a migraine headache is less common but more likely to send you to the doctor in quest of relief. Migraines occur more often in women than in men and can last from a few minutes to a few days. A third type, the cluster headache, is even more acute but also much more rare.

Whichever type of headache you're prone to, chances are that the underlying cause is your genetic makeup. "We are clearly dealing with a biological disorder, not a psychological one," says Fred Sheftell, M.D., a psychiatrist, headache specialist, and cofounder of the New England Center for Headache in Stamford, Connecticut. Still, there are things you can do to help yourself.

138

Pay attention to triggers. Just because you were born with a predisposition for headaches doesn't mean that you have to get them, according to Dr. Sheftell. If you can avoid the pain triggers, you might be able to avoid the headaches.

Heading up Dr. Sheftell's Top 10 list of triggers are sensitivities to foods such as chocolate, certain food components such as alcohol and caffeine, and the food additive MSG. Other possible triggers are hormone fluctuations during the menstrual cycle, changes in the weather or season, sleeping late or not enough, bright lights, and odors. And of course there's stress.

Traditional over-the-counter medications may get rid of the pain once it hits, but they won't help you have fewer headaches. With nutritional measures, you can take a preventive approach, says Dr. Sheftell.

Try riboflavin for migraines. In super-high doses, this B vitamin might ward off a migraine attack by helping the brain cells utilize energy, says Dr. Sheftell. That's because some people who get migraines may not have enough energy stored in their brain cells. Riboflavin helps the enzymes in the body tap into the energy stored in those cells.

Riboflavin is found in milk. Four glasses will give you the Daily Value of 1.7 milligrams. The doses needed to help prevent migraine are many times higher, however. "We start our patients on 200 milligrams for a week and then bring them up to 400 milligrams," Dr. Sheftell says.

According to Dr. Sheftell, some people experience nausea when they take as much as 400 milligrams. If that happens, you can just return to the 200-milligram dose. It may take some time to get relief, so stick with the supplements for 2 to 3 months before you decide whether they have any benefit, says Dr. Sheftell.

Add some magnesium. This mineral plays a key role in regulating both blood vessel size and the rate at which cells burn energy. Researchers estimate that 50 percent of migraine sufferers are magnesium deficient, says Burton M. Altura, M.D., professor of physiology and medicine at the State University of New York Health Science Center in Brooklyn. Does this mean that you can pop a few magnesium tablets to get rid of a headache? Not quite, but the supplement may be useful in preventing them.

"We believe that everyone should be taking 500 to 600 milligrams of magnesium a day in a combination of diet and supplements," says Dr. Altura. "If people brought up their total consumption of magnesium, they could reduce the frequency of recurring migraine headaches."

The trouble is, magnesium supplements often cause diarrhea, says Jacqueline Jacques, N.D., a naturopathic doctor and specialist in pain management in Portland, Oregon. This common side effect is a sign that the supplement is not being absorbed.

If you want to get the most from a magnesium supplement, Dr. Jacques advises taking magnesium glycinate instead of magnesium oxide or magnesium chloride. Magnesium glycinate is readily absorbed; it can go right to work and prevent constriction of the blood vessels in your brain and scalp, and since it is easily absorbed, it spends less time in the gut and is less likely to cause loose stools.

Feed on feverfew. A cousin of dandelion and marigold, feverfew has long been used to prevent headaches of all kinds. "It's important to understand that when you use a remedy preventively, it takes a fair amount of time to evaluate its effectiveness," says Dr. Sheftell. "You need to take 125 milligrams of feverfew every day for about 6 to 8 weeks."

Get pain relief from fatty acids. Try adding omega-3 essential fatty acids to your diet. Found in high amounts in fish oil and flaxseed oil, these key fats provide eicosapentaenoic acid (EPA), which changes your body chemistry so that your body produces fewer chemicals that increase sensitivity to pain and cause constriction of the blood vessels. Thus, you conquer the pain and also counteract the cause.

There's also a good chance that you'll get fewer migraines and less intense ones if you take 1 to 2 tablespoons of flaxseed oil every day, says Brent Mathieu, N.D., a naturopathic doctor in Boise, Idaho. Although you could see an improvement in as little as a few days, 4 to 8 weeks is more typical.

Flaxseed oil contains a substance that the body converts to EPA, so it is an indirect source of the important omega-3 fatty acid. "Fresh, cold-pressed flaxseed oil is the best natural source of omega-3 fatty acids," says David Perlmutter, M.D., a neurologist in Naples, Florida, and author of *Lifeguide*. For some people, however, fish oil may work better because it is a ready-made source of EPA.

If you take fish oil, take 1,000 to 2,000 milligrams a day in divided doses with meals, says Dr. Mathieu. The capsules sometimes cause unpleasant, fishy-tasting burping unless you take them with food.

Have an herbal moment. When your head is in the vise-like grip of a tension headache, take small doses of an herbal supplement that includes a mixture of valerian, passionflower, and skullcap, says Priscilla Evans, N.D., a naturopathic doctor at the Community Wholistic Health Center in Chapel Hill, North Carolina. This trio of herbs can help relax muscles in your shoulders, neck, and scalp. "Valerian is great for relaxing the nervous system, relieving tension, and providing general pain relief. Passionflower and skullcap help to calm stress," she says.

If you anticipate a stressful period that could trigger a tension headache, these soothing herbs can help minimize the impact. Stick with the manufacturer's recommendations if you choose a ready-mixed supplement. Typical instructions are to take 225 milligrams with meals or water twice a day. If you're using a tincture that combines the three herbs, take 10 drops three to four times a day, says Dr. Evans.

Go aspirin one better. For pain relief from tension headaches, use a supplement of white willow bark. This is the same salicylate-containing herb that led to the development of aspirin, says Dr. Mathieu. For effective relief, take one or two 400-milligram doses of dried bark capsules every 2 to 4 hours as needed.

"Willow bark is naturally buffered and acts gently, so it generally does not upset and irritate the stomach like aspirin," Dr. Mathieu says.

The herb also contains small amounts of vitamin C and quercetin and other bioflavonoids, which combine with the salicylate to relieve both pain and inflammation. The trade-off is that it's hard to regulate the dosage with herbs. "There's a wide variation in the quality of the plant and how it was prepared, so you never know exactly how much of the active substance you're getting," says Dr. Mathieu.

Although its active ingredients are less concentrated than the drugstore product, you shouldn't take willow bark if you are allergic to aspirin, says Dr. Mathieu.

Heartburn

You know the burning, painful feeling that occurs behind your breastbone whenever stomach acid flows back up from your stomach into your esophagus. And you're probably familiar with the over-the-counter antacid medications designed to relieve the symptoms. But these products don't cure heartburn.

While commercial antacids provide relief, many natural healers believe that we should try to do more than just reduce the acid. For one thing, it helps to improve your diet and digestion so the acid stays where it belongs—in the stomach. It also helps to use herbal and nutritional supplements that can heal the irritation and burning caused by any acid backup, says William Warnock, N.D., a naturopathic doctor in Shelburne, Vermont. Here's how to find relief.

Change your eating habits. Fatty, fried, or high-protein foods, alcohol, and coffee are often the culprits behind heartburn, says Pamela Taylor, N.D., a naturopathic doctor in Moline, Illinois.

People who gulp their food often get heartburn, says Dr.

Warnock. He advises eating regular meals and, above all, chewing food slowly.

Also, pay attention to the final meal of the day, suggests Dr. Taylor. "I tell patients not to eat within 4 hours of their bedtimes and that their last meal of the day should be oriented toward foods such as steamed vegetables, baked or broiled fish, and nonwheat grains such as rice or quinoa," she says.

Coat, soothe, and heal. Whatever the source of your heartburn, the mucous membranes of your esophagus are probably inflamed and irritated, says Melissa Metcalfe, N.D., a naturopathic doctor in Los Angeles. That's one area where supplements might be able to lend a helping hand.

An excellent herb to soothe those tissues is deglycyrrhizinated licorice (DGL), according to Dr. Metcalfe. DGL has antispasmodic action, which means that it helps to control various muscle actions that can affect your digestive tract. The herb also helps reduce acid reflux by calming a cramping stomach, she says.

The primary medicinal benefit of DGL, however, is its ability to increase and build up the protective substances that line the digestive tract. By stimulating the body's natural defense mechanisms, licorice helps prevent the formation of ulcers and lesions due to the irritating acid, says Dr. Metcalfe. It's also a powerful, localized anti-inflammatory. The typical dose is two 250-milligram capsules taken 20 minutes before mealtime.

Rather than swallowing the DGL with water, Dr. Metcalfe suggests that you suck on the capsules and let them dissolve slowly in your mouth. You can also get DGL in chewable tablets, which dissolve as you chew them. "You want the licorice to coat the inside of your throat and esophagus to cover those inflamed and irritated tissues," she says.

Use it for 4 weeks and then assess if it's working, she

suggests. If it is, your throat should feel less irritated. If not, see your health-care practitioner.

Get at the inflammation. Another healing substance for damaged mucous membranes is glutamine, an amino acid that's available as a nutritional supplement. Dr. Metcalfe frequently recommends it for gastrointestinal disorders whenever inflammation is a problem.

"I tell people to take one 500-milligram capsule four times a day until they feel better," says Dr. Metcalfe. "Usually, that's about a month."

Kill the bacteria. If bad bacteria—usually H. pylori—are the source of your problem, you could consider taking goldenseal, says Dr. Metcalfe. First, though, get a proper diagnosis from your doctor.

For best results, Dr. Metcalfe recommends that you combine a goldenseal supplement with colloidal bismuth, which is the active ingredient in many over-the-counter stomach medications like Extra-Strength Pepto-Bismol. Besides coating the stomach, the bismuth helps the herb adhere to the mucous membranes of the stomach.

Take two or three 400-milligram capsules of goldenseal daily along with 1 tablespoon of Extra-Strength Pepto-Bismol four times daily, Dr. Metcalfe suggests. "When you take bismuth, be aware that your stools will turn black. It's nothing to worry about." Don't use goldenseal if you are pregnant, however.

Get relief at the supermarket. Buy some ginger, says Dr. Taylor. Get either fresh ginger in the produce section or the powdered spice.

Ginger relaxes the smooth muscle along the walls of the esophagus, says Dr. Taylor. "If your digestion is working better, you're less likely to get that reflux, or backwash, of stomach acid," she says. "Ginger is an excellent tonic for the whole gastrointestinal tract."

If you're using ginger to prevent heartburn, take it 20 minutes before a meal. You can take it as a capsule, make a tea from the fresh root or the powder, or eat candied or pickled ginger as it comes from the jar. Ginger tincture is also available.

To use it in capsule form, take one or two "00" capsules and wait for a half-hour. If your symptoms don't improve in that time, you may repeat the dose. You can also empty the contents of the capsules into hot water, let it steep, and drink it as a tea, Dr. Taylor says.

Candied ginger has a long history as a digestive aid. Use a small amount, about the size of the tip of your little finger. Chew it slowly and well, incorporating a fair amount of saliva before swallowing, Dr. Taylor says. You can repeat this dose in 10 minutes or so if your symptoms have not lessened.

For tincture, she recommends a dose between 15 and 60 drops. "Always use the smaller amount, in a little water if possible. Repeat the 15-drop dose every 15 minutes, up to a total of 60 drops, if necessary."

Because ginger is considered a "hot bitter," people with very sensitive stomachs may find it too strong. If symptoms do not resolve with the above recommendations, consult your health-care practitioner.

Hip Pain

The last century hasn't been kind to the hip. From the hula hoop to hip-hop, boogie-woogie to break dancing, the joint has been jumping, bumping, and grinding at a mind-swiveling pace.

Yet these gyrations and dance sensations were hardly the hip's worst enemies. It's what Americans don't do in this increasingly sedentary age that really saps the zap from the hip.

"If anything, swinging your hips on the dance floor, walking to the post office, or just doing a few stretching exercises every day helps keep the muscles and bones of the joint strong. But we've gotten away from doing those things. The vast majority of Americans have become couch potatoes, and they're paying the price for it later in life in the form of thinner, weaker bones and an increased potential for hip fracture," says Jan I. Maby, D.O., director of the Geriatric Medical Home Care program at Mount Sinai Medical Center in New York City.

But it's never too late to make lifestyle changes, including regular exercise, to ease mild hip pain, strengthen weak bones, and reduce your susceptibility to hip fractures,

Dr. Maby says. In fact, many of the underlying causes of hip pain, such as arthritis, bursitis, and tendonitis, can easily be treated with these home remedies.

Seek the heat. Heat is one of your most potent allies against occasional hip pain, says Scott Marwin, M.D., vice chairman of the department of orthopedics at Long Island Jewish Medical Center in New Hyde Park, New York. Try placing an electric heating pad over your hip for 20 minutes three or four times a day, he suggests. If you don't have a heating pad, use a wet towel. Soak the towel in hot water and wring it out before applying it.

Give it ice. If heat isn't helping, apply ice where you feel hip pain to help reduce pain and swelling, says Craig Cisar, Ph.D., professor of exercise physiology at San Jose State University in California. To protect your skin, put a towel between your skin and the ice. Ice may be used for 15 to 20 minutes every 1 to 2 waking hours.

Reach for reliable relief. Over-the-counter extra-strength anti-inflammatory medications such as ibuprofen can reduce swelling and ease hip pain caused by arthritis, bursitis, and other muscle or joint injuries, says Jacob Rozbruch, M.D., orthopedic surgeon and assistant professor of medicine at Albert Einstein College of Medicine in New York City. If the recommended dosage on the label doesn't help, alert your doctor. You may have a hip fracture or another serious underlying problem that should be evaluated, he says.

Sidestep the ache. When getting out of a car, lift and swing both legs out of the door before standing, Dr. Marwin suggests. By rotating on your rear instead of twisting your pelvis, you'll lessen the strain on your back and hips. "If you step out of the vehicle one leg at a time, you put yourself into a spread-eagle position that is very aggravating to your hips," Dr. Marwin says.

Size up your assistance. A cane or walker is your best friend if it eases your hip pain and helps you stay independent, Dr. Maby says.

If you need a cane or walker for stability, be sure it is the right size, Dr. Marwin says. An ill-fitting assistive device will increase your hip pain, not relieve it. Ask your doctor to refer you to a medical supply store where you can be properly measured and outfitted with an appropriate cane or walker.

Be more able with a cane. When you use a cane, hold it in the hand opposite the injured hip, Dr. Marwin says. Move it forward at the same time that you step out with your injured hip, so you're distributing weight away from your bad hip and onto the cane. Then move your good hip forward as you take another stride.

Shed some pounds. Getting rid of excess body weight can help relieve the strain on your hips, Dr. Marwin says. In fact, each pound you lose will take 2 or 3 pounds of pressure off your hips.

"As you get older, it becomes more difficult for your muscles to offset your increased weight. As a result, your joints bear more and more of the brunt of the load, and they degenerate," Dr. Marwin says. "So keeping your weight down and staying physically fit are two of the best things you can do to preserve your hips."

Limber up. Stretching exercises often can relieve both hip and back pain by strengthening common muscles and increasing your flexibility, Dr. Rozbruch says.

Over time, Dr. Rozbruch says, loosening your hips will translate into more fluid, graceful, and pain-free movement. You can do the following stretches once a day to coax hip muscles into lengthening gently and slowly. But if you start to feel pain, stop. (And if you have a herniated disk, you should consult your doctor or physical therapist before trying any of these stretches.)

When to See a Doctor

- Pain radiates down into the groin.
- Your pain is caused by a fall or injury, even a minor one.
- The pain persists after a couple of weeks, despite self-care and home remedies.
- You can't bear weight on the hip.
- The pain occurs while you lie in bed at night or disrupts your sleep.
- You have difficulty walking or moving.
- You also have open sores on your feet or leg pain.

Lie down on a bed or on the floor on a mat, with your knees bent and your feet braced about 24 inches high on a wall, letting your head, upper body, and arms relax completely on the floor. (Hint: The farther from the wall you are, the easier this stretch will be.) You can support your head with a pillow or towel. Keep your buttocks on the floor. Keeping your right foot on the wall, cross your left foot over your right thigh, bringing the outer edge of your foot just below your right knee. If you are too stiff to reach that point, let your left leg cross farther over your right leg as much as needed.

Then, lift your right thigh toward your chest and reach your hands through to interlace around the back of the thigh. Create just the amount of stretch that is good for you by slowly drawing your right leg toward your chest. Hold for up to 1 minute. (If the reach is too difficult, use a towel to raise your thigh to your chest without lifting your head and shoulders off the floor.) Release and repeat on the other side. Note: You should feel this in the back of your left thigh, hip, or outer buttock, not in your lower back.

Another exercise: Lie down on your back on a bed or on the floor on a mat, with your legs extended and your feet wedged snugly and pressing against a wall. You can support your head with a pillow or towel. Make sure your toes point up toward the ceiling. On an exhalation, slowly draw your left knee toward your chest, interlacing your hands behind your knee/upper thigh. Hold this position for up to a minute, breathing evenly, then release. Repeat with your right leg. Avoid letting your straight leg bend and rise up. The most important part of this stretch is keeping one thigh pressed down onto the floor while you're flexing the other. Getting your knees to your chest is secondary.

Hot Flashes

Menopause is not really a single event but rather a process that can last a decade or longer. The average woman has her last period between the ages of 48 and 52, but menopausal changes actually begin much earlier. Women often notice changes in their cycles when they're in their early forties or even before then. Periods may be shorter or longer, lighter or heavier; they may come closer together or farther apart.

It's during this time, known as perimenopause, that the ovaries gradually slow their production of the female hormone estrogen and that a woman begins to notice the effects this has on her body. So why do some women experience such discomfort at menopause, while others never have so much as a single hot flash? It may be because some women experience more drastic drops in their estrogen levels than others do, says Margo Woods, D.Sc., associate professor of community health at Tufts University School of Medicine in Boston.

And some lucky women, about 25 to 30 percent, don't entirely stop producing estrogen, says Susan M. Lark,

M.D., director of the PMS and Menopause Self-Help Center in Los Altos, California, author of *Menopause: Self-Help Book*, and a physician specializing in women's health. Even after their ovaries stop producing estrogen, their adrenal glands and one small area of each ovary called the stroma continue to produce small amounts of this hormone. These glands don't produce enough estrogen to promote menstruation, but they do produce enough to keep the most bothersome symptoms of menopause at bay, explains Dr. Lark.

The amount of estrogen that the body continues to produce is out of your hands, adds Dr. Lark. But there are plenty of other factors you can control that can reduce menopausal discomfort. "Women who avoid stress, who don't overdo caffeine, and who get regular exercise have a much easier time of it," she says. Here are other things you can do to make the transition as comfortable as possible.

Snuff out hot flashes with vitamin E. A hot flash—that sudden, intensely hot feeling in your face and neck—can happen anytime, anywhere. Caused by hormonal surges, hot flashes usually last for 3 to 5 minutes, but they can feel like an eternity. Some women get flushed, sweat profusely, and even have heart palpitations. Other women have flashes so mild that they barely notice them. About 80 percent of all women going through menopause have hot flashes at one point or another.

Thin women are more prone to hot flashes than heavier women because, even after the ovaries slow their hormone production, fat cells continue to produce small amounts of estrogen. So women with a lot of fat cells go through less drastic estrogen withdrawal. While hot flashes can be relieved by hormone replacement therapy, there may be a less drastic option: a daily vitamin E supplement.

Make Healthy Diet Adjustments

Simple changes can make a big difference in your health during menopause, says Susan M. Lark, M.D., director of the PMS and Menopause Self-Help Center in Los Altos, California.

Shake the salt habit. Too much salt can contribute to water retention, a common problem among menopausal women, says Dr. Lark. Stop adding salt to your foods and eliminate fast foods, salty snacks, and other highly processed foods; use garlic and herbs instead of salt in cooking.

Switch to decaf. "Studies show that women who use caffeine have more hot flashes than those who don't," says Dr. Lark. Excess caffeine also increases anxiety, irritability, and mood swings and depletes the body's stores of B-complex vitamins. Eliminate caffeine gradually to avoid

Vitamin E can act as an estrogen substitute, explains Dr. Lark. Studies have shown that it can relieve hot flashes, night sweats, mood swings, and even vaginal dryness.

If you would like to try vitamin E, Dr. Lark recommends a fairly high dose: about 800 international units a day. And while vitamin E is nontoxic at this level, she says, women should get their doctors' okay before taking this high amount, especially if they have diabetes or high blood pressure.

Reduce bleeding with nutrients. Many women approach menopause expecting menstrual flow to taper off and finally stop. But for a good percentage, periods during perimenopause are heavier than ever and can seriously endanger their iron stores, says Dr. Lark.

Heavy bleeding can be treated effectively with nutrients, says Dr. Lark. "Some studies have shown that besides withdrawal symptoms like irritability and headaches. And don't forget that tea, chocolate, and cola drinks also contain caffeine.

Be a teetotaler. Alcohol depletes B-complex vitamins, disrupts the liver's ability to metabolize hormones, and can worsen hot flashes, says Dr. Lark. "Excessive drinking is also a risk factor for osteoporosis, which all menopausal women should be concerned about," she adds. Limit yourself to one or two drinks a week.

Eat more fruits and vegetables. Fresh produce is full of important vitamins and minerals, says Dr. Lark. And because they're low in fat and high in fiber, fruits and vegetables can help prevent weight gain, a common problem for women of menopausal age.

replenishing the iron lost through bleeding, a daily iron supplement may actually reduce the amount that a woman will bleed during future periods," she says.

Women with heavy bleeding also benefit from loading up on vitamin C and bioflavonoids, she says. Bioflavonoids are chemical compounds related to vitamin C; they're found in many citrus fruits and included in many supplements. Both reduce bleeding by strengthening the capillary walls, says Dr. Lark. And since bioflavonoids have many of the same chemical properties as estrogen, they can also be helpful in controlling hot flashes, night sweats, and mood swings. She recommends a daily supplement that includes at least 1,000 milligrams of vitamin C and 800 milligrams of bioflavonoids.

Because vitamin C helps the body absorb iron more efficiently, Dr. Lark recommends taking these two nutrients together. If you take a multivitamin/mineral supplement, check to make sure that it contains both vitamin C and iron. Another option is to take an iron supplement, about 15 milligrams, with a glass of orange juice. If you have a juicer, juicing the white pulp of the orange along with the rest of the fruit guarantees an abundant dose of bioflavonoids, Dr. Lark adds.

Battle the blahs with B complex. Depression is also common around the time of menopause, though nobody knows for sure how much of it results from hormonal fluctuations and how much is triggered by the everyday stresses of midlife.

Regardless of the cause, emotional stress can deplete the body of B vitamins, leaving a woman feeling tired, anxious, and irritable, says Dr. Lark. High levels of estrogen can also deplete vitamin B_6 and cause depression, she says.

Vitamin B_6 should always be taken as part of the B-complex, says Dr. Lark. She suggests a B-complex supplement containing 50 milligrams each of thiamin and niacin and 30 milligrams of B_6.

Cope with surgical menopause. Each year, thousands of women undergo hysterectomy, the surgical removal of the uterus and sometimes the ovaries because of conditions as varied as pelvic infection, endometriosis, and cancer.

In most cases, the woman's ovaries are left intact; they continue to produce estrogen until she goes through normal menopause. But if her ovaries are removed in a complete hysterectomy, she'll experience surgical menopause, with the same symptoms as any other woman who is going through natural menopause.

Women who experience surgical menopause may actually have more severe symptoms because they go through menopause so abruptly, says Dr. Lark.

A woman who undergoes a hysterectomy can benefit from the same nutritional strategies that help women who are going through natural menopause, says Dr. Lark. "As far as your body is concerned, it's the same process," she says.

Fight back with phytoestrogens. In Japan, hot flashes and night sweats are virtually unheard of. "Asian women and American women report such dramatically different experiences of menopause that it's easy to wonder if we're talking about the same thing," says Dr. Woods.

Researchers believe the traditional Japanese diet plays a role. Besides providing more vegetable protein and less animal protein than a Western diet, it's also low in fat and high in soy products such as tofu. These foods are rich in plant compounds known as phytoestrogens, which seem to mimic some of the biological activities of female hormones.

While the phytoestrogen content of soy foods varies considerably from brand to brand, one or two servings of tofu, soybeans, or soy milk a day is equivalent to the usual intake of the Asian population. It also contains approximately 35 milligrams of phytoestrogens, a reasonable goal to shoot for, says Dr. Woods.

Japanese women eat from 2½ to 3½ ounces of tofu per day, says Dr. Woods. "It can't hurt," says Dr. Woods. "Legumes, vegetables, and soy foods are safe, nutritious, and good for you, whether you're having hot flashes or not."

Insomnia

Anyone can have a sleepless night or two—or three. Before you reach for that over-the-counter sleeping pill or a prescription-strength remedy, however, consider some dietary and lifestyle changes to help catch up on your rest.

It's just common sense to eliminate caffeinated beverages and alcohol from your diet. Caffeine—whether from coffee, tea, or caffeinated soft drinks—is a nervous system stimulant that can keep you up at night. And alcoholic drinks disrupt the chemical messengers that help initiate sleep.

Moderate aerobic exercise, as long as you time it right, is good for improving sleep. Try to get at least 20 minutes of exercise a day in the morning or afternoon, but not right before bedtime. This might be enough to help you quickly fall asleep and stay asleep throughout the night.

If you still have insomnia after taking these steps, try these herbal and nutritional supplements.

Try valerian for steady sleep. This herb sends you off to dreamland quickly. Once you nod off, the deep sleep stages are deepened. What's more, you won't wake up as often during the night, nor will you feel fatigued and drowsy in the morning.

"Valerian root is a great herbal sleep aid because it sedates the central nervous system," says Chris Meletis, N.D., professor of natural pharmacology at the National College of Naturopathic Medicine in Portland, Oregon.

If anxiety, muscle tension, or muscle spasms leave you staring at the ceiling, valerian root can help relax these annoyances, says Thomas Kruzel, N.D., a naturopathic physician in Portland, Oregon.

Dr. Meletis recommends taking 400 to 425 milligrams of valerian root 1 hour before bedtime. "That will give the valerian plenty of time to wind down your nervous system," he says.

In some people, however, valerian acts as a stimulant, causing nervousness and heart palpitations. If this is the case, simply stop using it, advises Dr. Meletis. Also avoid valerian if you're taking sleep-enhancing or mood-regulating medications such as diazepam (Valium) or amitriptyline (Elavil).

Snooze with kava. Kava kava, another time-honored herbal insomnia fighter and muscle relaxant, can put you fast asleep if stress has been keeping you awake. Kava relieves anxiety and acts as a tranquilizer, says Kristy Fassler, N.D., a naturopathic doctor in Portsmouth, New Hampshire.

People who have taken kava for insomnia say that it continues to be effective over time, and it's not addictive. Also, it doesn't leave you feeling spaced-out or groggy the next morning as many of the prescription drugs do, says Dr. Fassler.

A 125-pound person should take two 150-milligram capsules, says Dr. Fassler. For each additional 30 pounds of body weight, add another 75 milligrams of kava, she advises. Kava begins working its magic pretty quickly, so take it about 20 minutes before bedtime. Do not take it if you are pregnant, breastfeeding, or trying to conceive.

Sleep Well with 5-HTP

A natural sleep aid has grabbed the attention of consumers. The pill is 5-hydroxytryptophan (5-HTP). It's an immediate precursor of serotonin, a vital brain chemical that regulates our moods, behavior, appetite, and sleep patterns.

Studies show that 5-HTP can shorten the time it takes to nod off and reduce middle-of-the-night awakenings. It is reported to increase the time you spend in REM sleep (the dream state) and in the deep sleep stages that you need to feel fully rested in the morning.

To fall asleep shortly after your head hits the pillow, take 25 to 50 milligrams of 5-HTP one hour before bedtime on an empty stomach or at least 2 hours after dinner, says Chris Meletis, N.D., professor of natural pharmacology at the National College of Naturopathic Medicine in Portland, Oregon.

Because 5-HTP may lose its effectiveness over time if you use it every night, take it only once or twice a week, says Ray Sahelian, M.D., a physician in Marina del Rey, California, and author of *5-HTP: Nature's Serotonin Solution*. It's advisable to consult your doctor before taking it, especially if you're taking prescription antidepressants, some of which interact with 5-HTP. The supplement has sedative effects that could be dangerous if you drive or operate heavy machinery, and high doses can cause nausea in some people. Women who are pregnant or trying to conceive should not take 5-HTP.

Pop some magnesium and calcium. Taken together, these two minerals act as mild muscle relaxants, says Dr. Meletis. Some research suggests that people who get less than 200 milligrams a day of magnesium can have shallow sleep patterns and more nighttime awakenings. These patterns of insomnia sometimes show up among people who have reduced their calorie intakes or have started on weight-loss diets.

Even if your magnesium intake is normal, certain medications such as diuretics for high blood pressure, which reduce water retention, cause the kidneys to excrete excessive amounts of the mineral. The Daily Value for magnesium is 400 milligrams from food and supplements, and this amount should be enough to prevent sleep problems. If you still have trouble sleeping, take 500 milligrams of magnesium and 500 milligrams of calcium, along with a carbohydrate like bread, within 1 hour of bedtime, says Dr. Kruzel.

Doze off with melatonin. Trumpeted as a panacea for jet lag, cancer, and depression, melatonin has been widely accepted for treating insomnia. This hormone is secreted by the pineal gland, a pea-size gland in your brain that helps control periods of sleepiness and wakefulness.

Before taking supplemental melatonin, have your doctor check your natural levels of melatonin. If they are low, take up to 1 milligram at least 2 hours before you go to bed, suggests Dr. Meletis. If you don't respond to this dosage, 2 or 3 milligrams may do the trick.

This supplement is for short-term use only. "Although melatonin works very well as a sleep aid, you shouldn't take it indiscriminately," Dr. Meletis says.

There hasn't been enough research to show whether there are long-term side effects from melatonin, he notes. It's possible that even at the recommended dosages, melatonin could disrupt your normal cycles of sleeping and waking, and other risks have also been associated with this supplement.

Irritability

Irritability sounds far too civilized to most Americans. So we invented slang like cranky, cross, crabby, vexed, and peeved. But no matter what you call it, occasional irritability is simply a part of being alive, says Laura Slap-Shelton, Ph.D., D.Ph., clinical psychologist with a specialty in neuropsychology at Jeanes Hospital in Philadelphia.

Irritability can go hand in hand with almost any illness, including anxiety, diabetes, and arthritis. And certainly, the aches and pains of later life can make us feel more irritable as the years and health problems begin to mount up, says George T. Grossberg, M.D., director of geriatric psychiatry at St. Louis University School of Medicine.

For those times when you feel mildly irritated, try these remedies.

Relax, then find the culprit. Whenever you feel irritable, take a few deep breaths and give yourself a mini-break in the action of the day, says Dr. Slap-Shelton. "You may want to take a walk or engage in your favorite form of exercise or your favorite hobby." Then, try to identify the culprit. Take a few minutes to think about what may be bothering you. Worry and fatigue often lead to irritability. If you can identify the cause of your irritability, especially a recurrent problem, it may help you banish it, Dr. Slap-Shelton says.

Take a break. Try engaging in a task that will distract you from whatever is irritating you, Dr. Grossberg says. Take a walk, dig in the garden, or make your bed. Even if the activity takes only 5 to 10 minutes, it will absorb your attention and give you time to cool off so you don't react impulsively or say something that you'll regret later.

Take a whiff. Oil of lavender can help relieve irritability, according to John Steele, a worldwide lecturer and aromatic consultant who runs Lifetree Aromatix, a company that sells botanical products and distributes information in Los Angeles. Apply three or four drops of the oil to a tissue or handkerchief and inhale whenever you feel irritable, he suggests. Lavender essential oil is the concentrated product of steam distillation. It is the most potent therapeutic part of the plant, says Steele. Essential oils are available at health food stores.

Send out warning signals. Let others know that you're having a bad day, Dr. Slap-Shelton advises. Simply admitting that things aren't going well and apologizing in advance for being out of sorts that day can help defuse the situation and bring about needed support and understanding.

"Often, people feel irritable because they feel overwhelmed by everything they need to do, and they don't know how to ask for support," Dr. Slap-Shelton says. Just say how you are feeling. "Friends and family will respond with empathy, humor, and other kinds of support that can go a long way toward getting you out of your bad mood."

Reach for the right foods. Fruits and vegetables are rich in complex carbohydrates, which increase serotonin, a brain chemical that produces an overall calming effect, says Julian Whitaker, M.D., founder and president of the Whitaker Wellness Center in Newport Beach, California. While it's always a good idea to eat plenty of produce, "when you're feeling irritable, it's especially important to eat more fruits and vegetables," he says.

Take a bath. A bath has a balancing effect on anxious or irritable people, according to Charles Thomas, Ph.D., co-author of *Hydrotherapy: Simple Treatments for Common Ailments* and a physical therapist at Desert Springs Therapy Center in Desert Hot Springs, California. Fill your bathtub with water slightly cooler than body temperature, around 94° to 97°F, according to Dr. Thomas. Submerging as much of your body as possible, he says, stay in the bath for at least 30 minutes, adding water as needed to maintain the temperature of the bath.

Image what's going on. Close your eyes and hear a silent cry from within. Feel this cry going out of you, says Elizabeth Ann Barrett, R.N., Ph.D., professor and coordinator of the Center for Nursing Research at Hunter College of the City University of New York in New York City. She suggests doing this imagery once a day in the morning as needed. It might take practice, she says, so if you don't feel the cry the first time, try again the next day.

When to See a Doctor

- Your irritability starts affecting your job performance and personal relationships.
- You have frequent or persistent headaches.
- Your irritability lasts for more than a week.
- You feel under constant pressure.
- You lose your appetite for 2 or more weeks.
- You withdraw from your usual activities.

As an alternative, imagine that your nerves are a series of stretched rubber bands throughout your body. One by one, release the rubber bands. Envision yourself relaxing more and more as each rubber band is released, says Dr. Barrett. She recommends that you do this imagery twice a day, once in the morning and once in the evening, and let it continue until you feel relaxed. If needed, she adds, you can repeat this imagery at any time during the day.

Relax and meditate. Meditation may help soothe irritability, says Sundar Ramaswami, Ph.D., a clinical psychologist at the F. S. Dubois Community Mental Health Center in Stamford, Connecticut. Use a picture, a word, an object (such as a candle flame), or a sensation (such as breathing) to focus your mind. If your mind begins to drift, refocus on the object. Begin meditating for 20 minutes twice a day, suggests Dr. Ramaswami. As you become more proficient and more aware of your body's sensations and needs, he says, you may find you can meditate less and still get the same effect.

Let music soothe your soul. Take a few minutes to imagine yourself swimming in a bubble of green light, says color-music therapist Mary Bassano in her book *Healing with Music and Color*. While you do this, listen to classical music such as Rubinstein's *Melody in F*, Debussy's *Clair de Lune*, or Mendelssohn's *Violin Concerto in E Minor*. Or try these New Age recordings: *Fairy Ring* by Mike Rowland or *Pan Flute* by Za Mir.

Try a supplement. A daily dose of an amino acid called gamma-aminobutyric acid, or GABA, can increase levels of the brain chemical serotonin, which has a calming effect and can help ease irritability, says Dr. Whitaker. You can buy GABA in supplement form in health food stores. Follow the manufacturer's suggested dosage on the label.

Jaw Problems

Jaw pain is very common, especially among people over age 60, says Paul A. Andrews, D.D.S., a dentist in Maitland, Florida, who practices therapeutic management of head, neck, and facial pain. "Often, jaw pain is a progressive problem that sneaks up on you."

Once your doctor has ruled out the possibility of a jaw fracture, the prime suspect will probably be TMD (temporomandibular disorder), which is an inflammation or misalignment of the joint that connects the jaw to the head. In studies, up to 75 percent of people have signs of TMD, including muscle pain and clicking, popping, or grating noises in the jaw, Dr. Andrews says.

Often, TMD and other forms of mild jaw pain are temporary and can be relieved by these simple home remedies, Dr. Andrews suggests.

Give your jaw a break. Treat your sore jaw as if it were a sore ankle, advises Flora Parsa Stay, D.D.S., a dentist in Oxnard, California, and author of *The Complete Book of Dental Remedies*. If your ankle were sore, you'd stay off it. The same rule applies to the jaw. While your jaw aches, try not to open it too wide. If you're a big yawner, that means you'll have to restrain yourself to avoid stretching your mouth too wide. But even when you're not yawning, you should be conscious of what position your jaw is in. Place your tongue on the roof of your mouth and keep your lips closed. That will help keep your teeth slightly ajar and keep your jaw in a relaxed position. Breathe through your nose. The only time your teeth should touch, Dr. Stay says, is when you are chewing or swallowing.

Hit it with an iceberg. Cold compresses can take the sting out of sore muscles surrounding the jaw, Dr. Andrews explains. Cold helps relax muscle spasms and numbs pain.

After you begin feeling pain, wrap an ice pack in a towel and hold it against your jaw for 20 minutes. Keep it off for 20 minutes, then apply the ice pack once more. Repeat as often as necessary to help ease the soreness.

Then melt it. If the pain persists for more than 36 hours, use a heat pack instead of a cold pack, following the same routine as you did when applying cold. The heat increases blood flow to injured tissues and helps them heal, Dr. Andrews says.

Toss the nuts. Avoid nuts, steaks, hard candies, caramels, and other chewy or crunchy foods when your jaw hurts, Dr. Andrews suggests. Stick with a soft diet that includes foods like macaroni and cheese, meat loaf, steamed vegetables, bananas, other tender fruits, juices, and water until the pain subsides.

Unplug the coffeepot. Caffeine increases muscle tension and makes the nervous system more sensitive to pain. So steer clear of coffee, teas, colas, chocolate, and other caffeine-laden beverages and foods if your jaw aches, Dr. Stay recommends.

Stoke up on C. Take vitamin C supplements. They'll help your body repair connective tissue surrounding the

When to See a Doctor

- Your jaw muscles feel tender and achy.
- You have a dull aching pain in front of your ear.
- You notice a clicking sound or grating sensation when you open your mouth or chew food.
- You have a persistent headache that seems centered behind your eyes.
- Your teeth or dentures don't come together normally.

jaw and hasten healing, Dr. Stay says. She recommends taking 2,000 milligrams of vitamin C daily. (Vitamin C in doses above 1,200 milligrams per day may cause diarrhea in some people.)

Use your noggin. Meditation may help relax muscles and relieve jaw pain, according to Dr. Andrews.

Focus on your breath as a simple, powerful way to meditate, he says. To try it, sit in a comfortable position, close your eyes, and take a couple of deep breaths. Inhale slowly through your nose for a count of 4, then slowly exhale through your mouth as you count to 10. Once you get accustomed to that pattern, stop counting breaths and focus all of your attention on the rhythm of your breathing as you inhale and exhale. To help you stay focused, try this: As you breathe in, think to yourself, "Calm mind." As you exhale, think, "Peaceful body." If your mind begins to drift, simply refocus your attention on your breath. Do this for 10 to 15 minutes a day or whenever your jaw pain seems worse, Dr. Andrews advises.

Glide into slumber. Devote your last waking hour each day to enjoyable activities like pleasurable reading, listening to soothing music, or soaking in a warm bath, suggests Gretchen Gibson, D.D.S., director of the geriatric dentistry program at the Veterans Administration Medical Center in Dallas. These routines will help relax your facial muscles and lessen the chances that you'll clench your teeth while you sleep.

"Don't do laundry, clean the kitchen, or take out the garbage at 9:45 P.M. and then hop into bed at 10:00. Your body won't be relaxed and you'll be more apt to wake up with jaw pain the next morning," Dr. Gibson says.

Straighten up and chew right. Poor posture forces your shoulders and head to pitch forward in order to maintain your balance, Dr. Andrews says. That can put extra strain on your jaw muscles and pull your teeth out of alignment, so chewing is more difficult.

To alleviate this problem, lie on a carpeted floor so that your back, shoulders, and the back of your head all touch the floor at the same time. Remain lying in that position for 15 to 20 minutes a day, Dr. Andrews suggests. If you like, you can prop your legs up on a pillow or chair.

Eyeball your dentures. Jaw pain can be a sign that your dentures are worn out and need to be replaced, Dr. Andrews warns. Check with your dentist.

Leg Cramps

Your nerves send signals to your muscles to tell them when to contract and relax. When these signals get scrambled, the muscle responds by cramping.

What mixes up the messages? The first suspected cause is a mineral imbalance, says Jacqueline Jacques, N.D., a naturopathic doctor and specialist in pain management in Portland, Oregon. That's not the only possibility, though. Cramps can also be caused by strenuous exercise, excess salt loss from sweating, or sitting or standing too long.

When you get a cramp, stretch and gently massage the muscle immediately. This should relax the muscle and provide you with some much-needed relief. If you find that you're having muscle cramps every night, your doctor is likely to prescribe quinine, but only for a limited time. This often-used treatment for leg cramps can quickly build to toxic levels in the blood and can cause nausea, vomiting, ringing in the ears (tinnitus), and deafness. It can even damage your eyesight.

A safer way to eliminate that knot of pain in your muscles is to try a combination of vitamin, mineral, and herbal supplements, say natural healers.

Reach for supplements. If you're getting a nightly wake-up call from your leg muscles, you probably need to get more magnesium and calcium, says Mark Stengler, N.D., a naturopathic doctor in Beaverton, Oregon, and author of *The Natural Physician: Your Health Guide for Common Ailments*. Both of these minerals are involved in relaxing nerve impulses and regulating muscle activity. Calcium is needed to contract the muscle, and magnesium is needed to relax it. An imbalance in this dynamic duo can irritate and confuse the muscle.

Since the calcium in bone provides a nearly inexhaustible mineral supply to replenish the relatively tiny amount that you need in your blood, you're more likely to be low on magnesium, says Dr. Jacques.

Mix in magnesium. If you're like most people, you probably get only 75 percent of the Daily Value (DV) for magnesium, which is 400 milligrams from food and supplements. Start with a dose of 250 milligrams of magnesium glycinate or chelated magnesium twice a day, says Dr. Jacques. These amino acid–based mineral supplements are easier to absorb than magnesium oxide. The more you absorb, the less likely it is that you'll have diarrhea, a common problem with magnesium supplements.

To help relieve cramps that interrupt your nightly sleep, take your second dose of magnesium right before you go to bed. If you don't get relief in 3 to 5 days, increase the dose to 500 milligrams twice a day, says Dr. Jacques. Stay at that level for another week to allow the tissue levels of the mineral to build up.

Take time for calcium. If cramps are still a problem at that dosage, add 500 milligrams of calcium to the regimen. The average adult absorbs only about 30 percent of the calcium consumed.

To maximize absorption, Dr. Jacques gives her patients calcium citrate instead of calcium carbonate, the form commonly found in antacid tablets. It helps to take it with a glass of milk since vitamin D is necessary for calcium absorption. If you are unable to drink milk, you can take a calcium supplement that also contains vitamin D.

If you're taking both calcium and magnesium, keep in mind that they work best when they are taken in certain ratios. The two ratios recommended by naturopathic doctors are either equal doses of calcium and magnesium or twice as much calcium as magnesium. Try the one-to-one ratio first, taking 500 milligrams of calcium and 500 milligrams of magnesium twice a day, Dr. Jacques says. If that doesn't give you the results you want, shift the ratio to 2:1 by reducing the magnesium to 250 milligrams.

Explore the E potential. Some patients with nighttime cramping have success with vitamin E, says Dr. Stengler. Although it has had mixed results in clinical trials, early studies suggest that you'll improve arterial blood flow and reduce leg cramping at night if you take vitamin E. To see if it works for you, take 400 to 800 international units a day, says Dr. Jacques.

Pump up your potassium. Potassium is another mineral that helps regulate muscle contraction, says Dr. Stengler. Deficiencies of this crucial electrolyte aren't normally a problem if you eat a variety of fruits and vegetables. If you change your diet drastically, however, you might become deficient. This is a potential problem if you go on one of the high-protein weight-loss diets that some experts advocate.

Cramps are more prevalent when you first start a high-protein diet, Dr. Jacques has observed. After a few months, they normally disappear on their own. To make them go away sooner, you can take one 99-milligram tablet of potassium a day, she suggests. This doesn't amount to much more than a bite or two of banana, but it can make your legs feel better, she says.

A word of caution, though: Don't take more than one tablet. It's easy to get too much potassium this way, which can upset the balance of other minerals in your body and cause heart and kidney problems. That's why Food and Drug Administration regulations don't allow more than 99 milligrams per tablet in over-the-counter supplements.

Don't ignore the little players. Maybe those cramps are due to an imbalance of trace minerals, especially if the pain is triggered by overexertion, says Dr. Jacques. You can deplete levels of trace minerals as you perspire. Electrolyte drinks (sports drinks) work well to help restore these depleted minerals. You can also take a trace mineral supplement that contains copper, manganese, zinc, selenium, and chromium, says Dr. Jacques.

Although trace mineral supplements vary in content, don't exceed the dosage guidelines on the bottle, she says. "Trace minerals should be taken in small doses because that's how they are found in your body. More is not better."

If you get leg cramps when you walk, see your doctor to rule out other conditions such as intermittent claudication, which is caused by poor blood flow to the legs.

Soothe spasms with herbal extracts. One of the most valuable is black cohosh (also known as black snakeroot, bugbane, and black cohosh root), says Dr. Stengler.

When muscles seize up with pain, take a 500-milligram capsule of the root powder or 30 to 60 drops of tincture in warm water every 1 to 2 hours.

For acute cramps, two or three doses should be sufficient for a therapeutic effect, says Dr. Stengler. Don't use black cohosh during pregnancy, though, or for more than 6 months at a time.

Bilberry has muscle-relaxant properties and helps to improve circulation in the extremities. To reduce muscle cramping, take 80 milligrams three times a day of an extract standardized to contain 25 percent anthocyanidin. You should take it for at least a couple of months, but you can continue indefinitely if necessary, says Dr. Stengler.

"Ginkgo is also useful, since it improves circulation through the extremities by dilating the arteries that feed the leg tissue," he says. While cramps are a problem, Dr. Stengler gives patients 60 milligrams three times a day of an extract containing 24 percent ginkgoflavoglycosides and 6 percent terpenelactones. If you have circulation problems, you can probably use ginkgo on a long-term basis.

Menstrual Cramps

Maybe you never thought about it, but if you add it up—month after month, year after year—you have your period for about 5 years of your life. And if you're like most women, you'd do anything to sail through those days without feeling crampy and exhausted and swollen up like a baby beluga.

Most women have some degree of menstrual discomfort at some point in their lives, says Susan M. Lark, M.D., director of the PMS and Menopause Self-Help Center in Los Altos, California, author of *Menstrual Cramps: A Self-Help Program* and *PMS: Self-Help Book*, and a physician specializing in women's health.

Most menstrual pain is classified as either spasmodic or congestive. Doctors know that spasmodic pain is caused by the female hormones estrogen and progesterone and by prostaglandins, hormonelike substances that control muscle tension. Women with spasmodic cramps generally have an excess of a certain type of prostaglandins called 2 series prostaglandins, which are responsible for contraction of the smooth muscles, including the uterus.

Prostaglandin production increases toward the end of your cycle, resulting in cramps that are sometimes accompanied by nausea, constipation, or diarrhea.

Probably the best thing that can be said about spasmodic pain is that it tends to improve with age. It's usually most severe in women in their teens and twenties. Spasmodic pain often improves after a woman has children, says Dr. Lark.

The other type of menstrual pain is known as congestive. Women with congestive pain also tend to suffer from bloating, water retention, headaches, and breast pain. In addition, they often notice a worsening of their cramps when they eat certain foods, such as wheat and dairy products, or when they drink alcohol, says Dr. Lark. Unfortunately, congestive pain tends to get worse with age, whether or not a woman has children.

While monthly cramps aren't pleasant, they are normal, says Dr. Lark. She cautions that in some cases, the pain can be a symptom of a health problem that requires medical attention, such as endometriosis. "You should always discuss unusual menstrual symptoms with your doctor," she advises.

But most of the time, the cause of cramps is simply menstruation itself. And in such cases, some doctors maintain that a few prudent nutritional changes can do wonders to improve your quality of life during your period, says Dr. Lark. The following nutrients have been shown to help soothe menstrual symptoms.

Give cramps a one-two punch. Getting enough of certain minerals all month long can make a significant difference in how a woman feels during her period. In one study, women reported much less severe symptoms when they followed a diet high in both calcium and manganese.

Just how these minerals fend off menstrual discomfort isn't clear. Researchers know that calcium is involved in the production of prostaglandins. "It may be calcium's role in prostaglandin metabolism that's responsible for the mineral's effect on pain," says James G. Penland, Ph.D., head researcher at the Grand Forks Human Nutrition Research Center in North Dakota.

Manganese's role is even more mysterious. "We do know that manganese is involved in blood clotting, and some research shows that a low intake is associated with a heavier menstrual flow," says Dr. Penland. "This is definitely an area that needs more study."

While researchers continue to try to figure out exactly how these two minerals work their magic on menstrual symptoms, a daily multivitamin/mineral supplement that includes the recommended levels of both calcium and manganese makes good sense for women who want to minimize menstrual discomfort, says Dr. Penland. The Daily Value for manganese is 2 milligrams. Because women of all ages have trouble getting enough calcium through diet, Dr. Penland recommends increasing your intake of low-fat, high-calcium foods such as low-fat yogurt and skim milk. If you still need more calcium, he suggests taking 500 to 1,000 milligrams of supplemental calcium a day.

Keep cramps at bay with vitamin B_6. The B-complex vitamins are essential for good health, but when it comes to relieving monthly symptoms, vitamin B_6 and niacin are the stars, says Dr. Lark.

Vitamin B_6 plays a key role in the production of "good" prostaglandins that relax the uterine muscles and keep cramps under control, according to Dr. Lark. But a woman's B_6 stores are easily depleted. Stress and certain medications, such as oral contraceptives, can easily cause a shortage. As a result, your body may not manufacture enough of the right kind of prostaglandins, leaving you feeling tied up in knots when your period comes. And if you're bothered by water retention or monthly weight gain, B_6 can ease those symptoms, too, Dr. Lark says.

Dr. Lark recommends taking vitamin B_6 as part of a B-complex supplement. Look for a B-complex supplement that contains no more than 200 to 300 milligrams of B_6. Large doses can be toxic, she says. It's a good idea to check with your doctor before taking doses of more than 100 milligrams daily.

Don't overlook niacin. Equally important in staving off cramps is niacin. "Some research shows that niacin is about 90 percent effective for relieving cramps," says Dr. Lark. To head off cramps before they start, she suggests

Foods That Ease Monthly Discomfort

How you feel during your period depends on what you eat during the rest of the month, says Susan M. Lark, M.D., director of the PMS and Menopause Self-Help Center in Los Altos, California. Here's what she advises.

Focus on fiber. Constipation is a common complaint of women with menstrual cramps, says Dr. Lark. Solve the problem naturally with a fiber-rich diet including plenty of fruits, vegetables, legumes, and whole-grain breads and cereals.

Banish wheat. Wheat can aggravate monthly symptoms in women who have food allergies, says Dr. Lark. If you suspect that you may be wheat-sensitive, substitute corn, oatmeal, brown rice, and rye bread for wheat products for a month or so to see if it helps.

taking between 25 and 200 milligrams of niacin a day, beginning 7 to 10 days before your period is due and stopping the day that your period starts. This treatment can be repeated every month to prevent menstrual cramps.

Because niacin can cause slight flushing in some women, start with 25 milligrams a day for the first month. "If it doesn't seem to help, you can always increase the dose the following month until you find the level that's right for you," she advises. Women with liver disease should use niacin only under medical supervision, cautions Dr. Lark.

Lessen bleeding with the right nutrients. Next to cramps, heavy bleeding is probably the most common complaint of menstruating women, says Dr. Lark. Besides being inconvenient, heavy bleeding can deplete a woman's iron stores and can even lead to anemia.

Steer away from beef. A diet high in red meats such as beef, lamb, and pork may aggravate menstrual cramping, says Dr. Lark. Meats contain saturated fat, which the body uses to produce chemicals that are responsible for the contraction of the smooth muscles of the uterus, which leads to cramping, she explains.

Beware of hidden sodium. Too much salt in the diet can aggravate monthly water retention, says Dr. Lark. Much of the salt you eat is hidden in seemingly healthy foods, such as canned vegetables, frozen dinners, and cheeses. Fast foods, pizza, and most snacks are also heavily salted. Don't add salt at the table and during cooking. Read labels for sodium content; salad dressings, prepared soups, and many condiments are loaded.

It isn't surprising, then, that doctors recommend iron supplements to women with heavy bleeding. What is surprising is that getting extra doses of this mineral doesn't just replace the iron that has been lost. It may actually reduce the amount of bleeding in the future, says Dr. Lark.

"Women need only a small amount of iron. But what they need they really need," she says. She recommends a daily supplement of about 15 milligrams.

Women with heavy bleeding also need plenty of vitamin C and bioflavonoids, says Dr. Lark. Bioflavonoids are chemical compounds related to vitamin C; they're found in many citrus fruits and included in many supplements. Both vitamin C and bioflavonoids reduce bleeding by strengthening the capillary walls, which are at their weakest just before and during the menstrual period, says Dr. Lark. She recommends a daily supplement that includes at least 1,000 milligrams of vitamin C and 800 milligrams of bioflavonoids.

Because vitamin C helps the body absorb iron more efficiently, Dr. Lark recommends taking these two nutrients together.

Mood Swings

For some people, it doesn't take much to change their moods: a song on the radio, the color of the walls, their spouse's voice telling them good night. And in some cases, the mood swings are legendary, shifting faster than an Indy 500 driver.

What causes such swings? In women, mood swings are often related to hormonal fluctuations and may occur before the monthly period, during and right after pregnancy, and during menopause. But female hormones aren't the only culprits: Men, too, can go into funks—over a cloudy sky, a spouse's offhand comment, or just a stressful day at work. Thankfully, there are natural ways to help control mood swings, say some health professionals.

Say no to certain foods. "When people have an overgrowth of yeast in their intestines, they can have a lot of emotional shifts, because certain substances are released into their blood that affect their psyches," says Elson Haas, M.D., director of the Preventive Medical Center of Marin in San Rafael, California, and author of *Staying Healthy with Nutrition*. Other people develop emotional reactions to certain foods, such as refined sugar, he says. If you're prone to mood swings, he recommends limiting your intake of yeast-producing foods such as vinegar and baked goods as well as of refined sugar, caffeine, and alcohol.

"Mood swings can also be caused by foods that typically cause allergic reactions in people—things such as milk products and wheat," says Dr. Haas. "So if you notice mood swings after consuming these foods, you might have a food allergy and should avoid them."

Take a soak. A bath is a classic treatment for emotional ups and downs, says Tori Hudson, N.D., a naturopathic physician and professor at the National College of Naturopathic Medicine in Portland, Oregon. The next time you need to chill out, fill your tub with water just slightly cooler than body temperature. It should feel like a hot bath that's beginning to get a little chilly, says Dr. Hudson. Soak for 20 minutes, adding water as needed to maintain the temperature of the bath.

Get juiced. "Mood swings are often caused by problems in the pancreas," says Eve Campanelli, Ph.D., a holistic family practitioner in Beverly Hills, California. "Carrot juice contains natural insulin and stabilizes the pancreas." Many people may be able to control mood swings by minimizing the amount of sugar in their diets and by drinking two glasses of fresh carrot juice a day, according to Dr. Campanelli. Because carrot juice is quite sweet, she recommends diluting 4 ounces of the juice with an equal amount of water for each glass.

Soothe yourself with music. Mood swings may arise because of stress, anger, or anxiety, says Janalea Hoffman, R.M.T., a composer and music therapist based in Kansas City, Missouri. Some people find relief from shifting moods by listening to relaxing music with a slow, steady beat, which slows your heart rate and calms your mind, she says. Try listening to this type of music for about 30

When to See a Doctor

- Your sleep patterns are disturbed.
- Your mood swings are unpredictable, uncontrollable, or inappropriate to the situation.
- Your moods alternate between intense joy and deep despair.

minutes a day. She suggests her tapes *Musical Hypnosis* and *Deep Daydreams*. Other good choices include compositions by Bach, Vivaldi, and Handel.

Listen to the ocean. If you live near the ocean, try sitting on or near the beach for a half-hour or so each day. Ocean waves crash the shore at a steady rhythm that helps calm you down, Hoffman says. "That's why people feel so good at the ocean," she says. "It's a constant sound, a relaxing sound. And people really respond to the rhythm."

If you can't get near the ocean, Hoffman suggests buying or making a tape recording of ocean waves. "It's probably not quite as good as the real thing, but the rhythm will still be the same," she says. You can find these tapes in many music stores. But, she adds, the sound of real waves is better than synthesized waves.

Muscle Cramps

Muscles are the foot soldiers of the human body. Some, such as the heart, are independent. But more than 600 others bend and stretch to accommodate our every whim.

Only when we've forced them to do something ridiculous do muscles make their presence known, often in the form of muscle cramps, which are painful, spasmodic muscular contractions. Cramps often mean you've spent too long in an unnatural position: sitting in a cramped car for several hours or sleeping in a position fit for a circus contortionist. Muscle pain can mean you've pushed your body too far, whether in a vigorous game of touch football or by attacking the weeds in your garden like a Tasmanian devil. The natural remedies in this chapter may help prevent or relieve muscle cramps, according to some health professionals.

Try a fragrant massage. To relieve your aching muscles, Los Angeles aromatic consultant John Steele suggests a blend of anti-inflammatory essential oils: three drops of blue chamomile, three drops of birch, three drops of rosemary (or coriander), eight drops of lavender, three drops of ginger (or black pepper), and ½ ounce of a carrier oil such as olive, almond, grape seed, or avocado. (The oils are available in health food stores.) Massage into the affected area after a warm bath, says Steele.

Get your feet wet. To stop muscle spasms, soak your feet for 10 to 20 minutes in a large pot of hot water with a homemade tea bag of black or brown mustard seeds (2 teaspoons of seeds tied up in some cotton or cheesecloth) immersed in it, says Vasant Lad, B.A.M.S., M.A.Sc., director of the Ayurvedic Institute in Albuquerque, New Mexico. Mustard seeds are available in health food stores.

Eat your vegetables. And have them raw, since cooking them depletes their potassium, magnesium, and calcium, the three nutrients most important in preventing and treating muscle cramps and pain, says Julian Whitaker, M.D., founder and president of the Whitaker Wellness Center in Newport Beach, California. "Eating foods rich in potassium and magnesium is the best thing for muscle cramps," he says. Potatoes, bananas, and dried fruits are

When to See a Doctor

- You have cramps several times in 1 day or cramps that "lock" for several minutes.
- Your muscle pain is accompanied by a fever or tender areas in the neck, shoulders, back, chest, hips, and buttocks.
- You have a muscle spasm in your back or neck that causes weakness, numbness, or tingling.
- You have a muscle spasm that doesn't improve within 3 days.

high in potassium. Nuts, wheat germ, and pumpkin seeds are good sources of magnesium. Low-fat dairy products and salmon and sardines with their bones have lots of calcium.

Have an herbal massage. For massaging out muscle tension, Mary Bove, L.M., N.D., a naturopathic physician and director of the Brattleboro Naturopathic Clinic in Vermont, recommends this herbal massage oil. Start with 1 cup of extra-virgin olive oil or almond oil. Add the following herbs in tincture form: 1 ounce of cramp bark, ½ ounce of lobelia, and ¼ ounce of willow bark or wintergreen. (If you don't have wintergreen tincture, Dr. Bove says to substitute 30 drops of wintergreen oil.) These ingredients are available in health food stores.

Stay cool. A frozen bandage is great for minor sprains, minor sports injuries, and spasms that do not respond to heat, says Agatha Thrash, M.D., a medical pathologist and cofounder and codirector of Uchee Pines Institute, a natural healing center in Seale, Alabama. Dip a hand towel in very cold water, squeeze it out, place it in a plastic bag, and store it in the freezer over a piece of cardboard, so the towel freezes flat. To use, remove the plastic and lay the bandage over the affected area. The rigid bandage will quickly become soft as it's warmed by your body heat. Replace with a fresh bandage when the towel feels warm. Dr. Thrash recommends 20-minute sessions of this treatment two to four times a day for a week or until symptoms subside.

Imagine yourself pain-free. Close your eyes, breathe out three times, and imagine your muscle encased in a block of ice, writes New York City psychiatrist Gerald Epstein, M.D., in his book *Healing Visualizations*. Picture the ice melting, and as it melts, feel the muscle relax. After the ice has completely melted, open your eyes, and the muscle spasm or cramp should be gone.

Dr. Epstein suggests doing this imagery for 2 to 3 minutes as needed every 15 to 30 minutes until the pain subsides.

Massage yourself. Run your fingertips very lightly up and down the length of the affected muscle, says Vincent Iuppo, N.D., naturopathic physician, massage therapist, and director of the Morris Institute of Natural Therapeutics, a holistic health education center in Denville, New Jersey. Use long, gliding strokes and make sure they're gentle, as if you were running a feather duster over the muscle. Continue until the pain or cramp has subsided.

Practice a relaxation routine. Whenever muscle cramps put a crimp in your day, reduce them with this stretch-based relaxation technique, says Charles Carlson, Ph.D., professor of psychology at the University of Kentucky in Lexington.

Push up your eyebrows with your index fingers and push down on your cheeks with your thumbs. Hold for 10 seconds. Release and let the muscles relax for a minute. Let your head slowly drop toward your right shoulder for 10 seconds, then toward your left shoulder for 10 seconds. Don't raise your chin.

Put your hands together as if praying. Keeping your fingertips and palms together, spread your fingers. Move your thumbs down along the midline of your body until you feel a light stretch in the lower arms. Hold for 10 seconds, then relax.

Interlock your fingers and raise your hands over your head. Straighten your elbows and rotate your palms outward. Then let your arms move back over your head until you feel resistance. Hold for 10 seconds, then release and let your arms rest at your sides.

Nausea

Nausea is not a disease. From your body's point of view, it's not even a problem but a safety mechanism. Nausea usually strikes as a kind of distress signal. If you swallow something that your digestive system doesn't like or that it even suspects is bad for you, it sends out an alarm through the complex system of nerves that connects your stomach to your brain.

If your body is experiencing other stresses like motion sickness, emotional distress, or even unpleasant sights or odors, your body may again use this distress signal to get your attention and register a problem. And it's an effective signal. Say what you want about nausea, but it's certainly hard to ignore.

If you've long suffered from problems like motion sickness or the nausea that sometimes accompanies migraine headaches, you're all too familiar with the conditions that may be your nemesis. But there can be other causes.

Medication is a common cause of nausea, says Robert Charm, M.D., gastroenterologist and internist in Walnut Creek, California, and professor of gastroenterology and internal medicine at the University of California, Davis. Sometimes, you may simply be sensitive to one type of medicine. Or a combination of different medicines may be interacting to make you ill.

Even if the cause isn't obvious, there are ways to spot the source of your nausea and ease that queasy feeling whenever it strikes—especially if it's caused by a motion that your body doesn't like.

Take a break. Your tummy will feel calmer if you rest a bit when a wave of nausea hits. Put your feet up and sit a spell. If you're in a car, pull over, roll down the window, and get some air. While you're resting, gaze out the window, says Roger L. Gebhard, M.D., gastroenterologist at the Veterans Affairs Medical Center and professor of medicine in the division of gastroenterology at the University of Minnesota, both in Minneapolis. "People with nausea often feel better if they can look outside and focus on the environment."

Change your meal plan. In the midst of a nausea spell, don't eat anything. Wait a couple of hours in order to give your stomach time to settle, says Dr. Charm.

Give nausea the sip. If you have nausea, sip—don't gulp—some clear liquid. Flat soda, water, a fluid replacement drink like Gatorade, and some clear broth are all good choices. Take a sip once or twice every 5 minutes, suggests Dr. Charm. Hydration is especially important if you are also experiencing vomiting, he says.

Snack a little. If the nausea has passed and you haven't eaten anything for a couple of hours, then it's okay to eat something light. Just be sure to make it a low-fat snack of plain foods. Spicy and fatty foods are hard to digest and can make a queasy stomach feel even worse. "Some white rice, toast, or crackers can help," says Martin Brotman, M.D., a gastroenterologist at California Pacific Medical Center in San Francisco.

When to See a Doctor

- The nausea lasts more than 3 days for no apparent reason. (It could be the first sign of a heart attack or indicative of ulcers or problems of the gallbladder, liver, or pancreas.)

Swallow some relief. Pepto-Bismol, Mylanta, or other over-the-counter antacids can help calm an unsettled stomach.

For nausea linked with dizziness and motion sickness, take dimenhydrinate (Dramamine). But be aware that motion sickness medicines won't do much good if the nausea is from the flu or something you ate, says Dr. Brotman.

Chew on some ginger. For a natural nausea reliever, chew candied crystallized ginger, which you can find in natural food stores or the spice aisle of your supermarket.

Or add some fresh ginger to your meals. "Grate the ginger into sauces or food, such as chicken," says Mike Cantwell, M.D., clinician and coordinator for clinical research at the Institute for Health and Healing at the California Pacific Medical Center in San Francisco. "You can also make ginger tea."

Press here. If your nausea comes from motion sickness, you may be able to relieve it with an acupressure wrist band (Sea-Band), which is specially designed to apply pressure to a pressure point on the inner wrist that can actually help ease nausea. You'll find these bands in some drugstores and in the sporting goods area of some department stores.

Nosebleed

Dog owners know that a moist nose is a healthy nose. The same is true for people, mostly. We don't have slippery, leather-like muzzles on the ends of our faces, but our noses produce a lot of moisture, about a quart of mucus a day, says Louis D. Lowry, M.D., professor of otolaryngology at Thomas Jefferson University Hospital in Philadelphia. The mucus, which is about 95 percent water, humidifies the air we breathe for the lungs.

As we get older, though, that moisture in our noses can dry up. The delicate membrane inside becomes dry and brittle, exposing a delicate network of veins and arteries that can break open and cause a nosebleed at even the slightest sneeze or sniff.

Unless they last for a long period of time, nosebleeds aren't terribly serious, but they are annoying and a little scary. You can stop or prevent them with these simple measures.

Stem the flow. There are three basic steps to follow to stop a nosebleed, says Jack B. Anon, M.D., otolaryngologist at Peach Street Medical in Erie, Pennsylvania, and chairman of the Nasal and Sinus Committee for the American Academy of Otolaryngology–Head and Neck Surgery.

1. Sit up straight with your head tilted slightly forward so that the blood doesn't run down your throat.
2. Gently blow out of your nose any clots that could prevent a blood vessel from sealing.
3. Put the squeeze on. Pinch the soft part of your nose between your thumb and forefinger for 10 minutes. "Sometimes, people don't know where to squeeze. The nose is designed so that your fingers fit right in the soft part on the outside of your nose," says Dr. Anon. Some blood will come out when you squeeze—but just hold a folded-up tissue at the base of your nostrils to catch the drips.

Spray the vessels shut. If your nose does not stop bleeding after 10 minutes of steady squeezing, use a nasal spray, such as Afrin or Neo-Synephrine, to constrict the vessels in your nose and stop the blood flow. Put four or five squirts in the bleeding nostril and pinch the soft part of your nose for an additional 10 minutes, says Dr. Anon.

Don't dry out. If you are developing nosebleeds from a dry nose caused by a lack of mucus production, moisten the membrane in your nasal passage with a saline spray to prevent it from cracking and rupturing. Spray the saline in your nose in the morning and evening, says Dr. Lowry.

Humidify your home. Breathing heated air in the winter or cooled air in the summer can dry out your mucous membranes and make you more prone to nosebleeds. Use a cool-mist humidifier to add moisture back into the air and your mucous membranes, says Dr. Lowry. To make sure the level of moisture in your home stays at or above

When to See a Doctor

- Your nose does not stop bleeding after 20 minutes of applying pressure.
- You feel blood running down the back of your throat when you are sitting or standing up or after you have pinched your nostrils.

40 percent relative humidity, buy a gauge at a home-electronics store like Radio Shack.

Avoid heavy lifting or bending. Although direct pressure on the blood vessels will make them stop bleeding, pressure from within the vessels will start the flow again, says Dr. Anon. Avoid straining the vessels by lifting anything heavy. And keep your head above the level of your heart to avoid putting pressure on the vessels.

Take your vitamins at night. If you are prone to nosebleeds, be sure you are getting enough vitamin C, which is important in the maintenance of the blood vessels, and vitamin K, which is necessary to control bleeding. The Daily Values are 60 milligrams for vitamin C and 80 micrograms for vitamin K. To get the most out of nutritional supplements, you should take them at night, says John A. Henderson, M.D., otolaryngologist and assistant professor of surgery/otolaryngology at the University of California, San Diego, School of Medicine.

"Take your nutritional supplements at bedtime. If you take them at breakfast, they'll be in the urine within 7 minutes," he explains. "Your kidneys slow down when your body is horizontal and sleeping, and vitamins will remain in your system longer and be absorbed."

Overeating

First, an irresistible urge compels you to eat large amounts of food in one sitting. Days later, you're at it again, wolfing down bagfuls of whatever you can get your hands on. Extreme feelings of guilt and distress follow each episode, but even that doesn't stop you from repeating this uncontrollable eating pattern over and over again.

If this sounds familiar, you might be among the one to two million Americans who have binge-eating disorder. The hardest part may be looking for help.

When you are used to hiding a problem like this, it's extremely difficult to tell anyone about it—even your own doctor. Nevertheless, the first thing you should do is see your physician. You need to be diagnosed—and to find out what your treatment options are—before taking any nutritional supplement, says Nancy Dunne Boggs, N.D., a naturopathic doctor in Missoula, Montana.

Most of those who have binge-eating disorder are obese, and the condition is slightly more common in women, affecting three women for every two men. What's more, binge eating is the most prevalent eating disorder among

African-American women, which may explain why they're twice as likely as white women over 30 to be obese.

Research shows that mild to moderate depression is the most common cause, says Dr. Boggs, so it's important to treat the depression with medication and counseling. Practitioners of alternative medicine say one of the best ways to treat the depression associated with binge eating is to take a variety of nutritional supplements—they can increase the levels of certain brain chemicals, or neurotransmitters, that lift your mood, suppress your appetite, and eliminate cravings.

Bring in the Bs. Because binge eaters tend to consume large quantities of high-fat foods that have little or no nutritional value, many are deficient in important B-complex vitamins and the minerals chromium, magnesium, and zinc, says Susan Kowalsky, N.D., a naturopathic doctor in Norwich, Vermont.

The B vitamins are needed to manufacture important brain chemicals, such as serotonin, that are responsible for regulating your moods, emotions, sleep patterns, and appetite. Vitamin B_6, in particular, helps convert the amino acid tryptophan to serotonin in your brain, says Dr. Kowalsky. Serotonin is a chemical messenger that has been closely associated with many emotional states, including depression.

Vitamin B_{12} helps other neurotransmitters work together to relieve depression. In addition, this vitamin helps your body make use of other mood-elevating brain chemicals such as dopamine and norepinephrine.

Dr. Kowalsky suggests taking a high-quality B-complex multivitamin daily. These may be labeled as B-50 or B-100 complex multivitamins, depending on whether they contain 50 or 100 milligrams of the B vitamins that are listed on the label. Many brands are available.

Mind your minerals. Chromium and magnesium can help eliminate cravings and stabilize levels of blood sugar (glucose), which fluctuate wildly when a person binges on large amounts of food, says Dr. Kowalsky.

Take 200 micrograms of chromium and 500 to 700 milligrams of magnesium daily, says Dr. Kowalsky, but be sure to check with your doctor first if you have heart or kidney problems.

And supplementing with zinc can help derail your appetite by activating a brain signal that tells you when you're hungry and when you're full. Dr. Kowalsky recommends taking 15 milligrams of zinc daily. If you take a multivitamin, you're probably getting all you need, since that's the amount found in most multis.

Boost serotonin with 5-HTP. Binge eaters commonly produce low levels of serotonin, so their appetites become ravenous. They tend to crave high-fat carbohydrates and are less likely to receive a signal telling them that they're full.

That's where 5-hydroxytryptophan (5-HTP) can help. Shortly after you take 5-HTP in supplement form, the compound travels to your brain and is converted to serotonin. The boost in serotonin suppresses your appetite. You'll be in better spirits, your binge eating will be under control, and you'll eventually lose weight, says Dr. Boggs.

She suggests taking 50 milligrams of 5-HTP three times a day. If you don't notice any decrease in your cravings and binge eating after 6 weeks, take 100 milligrams three times a day. If there is still no improvement after 6 weeks, increase to 200 milligrams three times a day, but don't exceed 900 milligrams daily. You can find this supplement in health food stores. Be sure you don't take it with other medications, especially antidepressants, unless you talk to your doctor.

Break the cycle with St. John's wort. Like 5-HTP, this herb raises serotonin levels in the brain, but its action is different.

Researchers speculate that St. John's wort may inhibit the enzyme called monoamine oxidase, which breaks down serotonin molecules and other brain chemicals. Or perhaps it increases the action of serotonin at the nerve endings in the brain. (A number of pharmaceutical antidepressants work this way, too.) Attached to the receptor sites in your brain, the serotonin helps to boost your mood, stabilize your appetite, alert you when you're full, and prevent binge-eating episodes.

To get the benefits of St. John's wort, Dr. Boggs suggests taking 300 milligrams two or three times a day with meals. Look for a standardized extract containing 0.3 percent hypericin.

Rashes

Lots of things cause rashes—plants, pets, jewelry, rubber, perfume, and fungi, to name a few. And if you've brushed up against poison ivy or developed athlete's foot after using the shower at the local swim club, you know where the rash came from.

Many times, however, a rash seems to appear out of nowhere. When the skin comes in contact with an allergic substance, the reaction is not immediate. A few days may pass before the rash takes hold—though once you have it, the rash can last a week or longer.

One way to figure out the cause is to look at the location. If the rash is caused by an internal trigger like food, medication, or virus, the rash will generally be more widespread and symmetrical. If something external like detergents or poison ivy caused the rash, it will be confined to areas of the skin that were exposed to the irritant, says Patricia Farris Walters, M.D., clinical assistant professor of dermatology at Tulane University School of Medicine in New Orleans.

Allergies may also be the problem and can develop at any age. Plus, if you've moved to a new location, you may find yourself exposed to a new allergy problem. Most rashes need to be looked at by a dermatologist if they last longer than 2 to 3 days. But meanwhile, you'll want some methods to soothe the irritation, itching, and inflammation. Here they are.

Cool with creams. An over-the-counter corticosteroid cream may provide relief from itching, burning, and irritation, says Thomas Fisher, M.D., a dermatologist in private practice in Chicago. He says that application of 1-percent hydrocortisone applied thinly four times daily should provide some relief.

Or try an antibiotic ointment containing polymyxin bacitracin twice daily with hydrocortisone, Dr. Fisher recommends. Avoid over-the-counter ointments with neomycin, since it can cause allergic reactions.

Cool it. If a rash starts oozing, Dr. Fisher recommends a cool compress with aluminum subacetate—Burrow's solution. You can make Burrow's solution from effervescent tablets that are sold in pharmacies as Domeboro.

To make a compress, soak a clean handkerchief or piece of gauze in Burrow's solution, then place the damp cloth on the affected area for 5 minutes. Repeat this process four times for a total 20-minute session. Do this 20-minute treatment three times daily. Follow each treatment with medicated cream.

Try a hot rinse. The itch of poison ivy can be turned off for extended periods by running hot water over the affected area, says Andrew T. Weil, M.D., director of the program in integrative medicine and clinical professor of internal medicine at the University of Arizona College of Medicine in Tucson. For 5 to 10 minutes, rinse the area with water that's as hot as you can stand without risk of burning yourself, he says. At first, the hot water will increase the itch, but after a few minutes, "the nervous circuits seem to get overloaded and the itching stops for a long time," he says.

When to See a Doctor

- Your rash is accompanied by dizziness, nausea, or difficulty breathing.
- You have a rash for longer than 2 to 3 days.

Soak in soda. A half-cup of baking soda in a tub full of bathwater makes a rash-relieving soak. "You could also make a paste from a spoonful of baking soda mixed with a bit of water and dab that on your rash to soothe your skin," says Dr. Walters.

Soothe with salves. As an alternative to cortisone, Dr. Weil suggests calendula cream, made from the petals of a marigold-like flower that is prized for its healing effect on skin. Calendula cream is available in health food stores.

Cover with care. Ordinarily, you leave a rash uncovered, says Dr. Walters, but if it's wet, oozing, and blistering, you may want to cover it with a light gauze bandage to prevent an infection.

Take an antihistamine. To reduce swelling and itching, take a nonprescription antihistamine, like diphenhydramine (Benadryl), at bedtime, suggests Andrew P. Lazar, M.D., associate professor of clinical dermatology at Northwestern University Medical School in Chicago. Benadryl may make you drowsy, which can be an added benefit if the itch has been keeping you awake at night, he says. Before taking an antihistamine, however, be sure to check for any interaction with your prescription drugs, cautions Dr. Lazar. Some antihistamines can speed up your heart rate. For someone with an enlarged prostate, an antihistamine might impede urination.

Restless Legs

When you—and your legs—are ready to rest, restless legs are ready to run. Sensations of jumpiness, itchiness, burning, aching, or twitching are all common in people with restless legs.

"It's often an unrecognized cause of insomnia," explains Jay Lombard, M.D., assistant clinical professor of neurology at Weill Medical College of Cornell University in New York City and co-author of *The Brain Wellness Plan*. You may think that you "just can't sleep," but in fact, it's the annoyance of your overactive limbs that is robbing you of your rest.

Calming restless legs can require some patience. If you're a pregnant woman, your legs will probably feel better after you've had your baby. Smokers with restless legs should quit smoking to give their leg circulation a chance to flow full force. For some people with severe restless legs, a trial of medication may be in order. Then, there are also some leg-soothing supplements that are definitely worth trying.

Calm cranky muscles with a mineral trio. A combined deficiency of three minerals could be responsible for the annoying jumpiness of restless legs syndrome, according to

Ross Hauser, M.D., director of Caring Medical and Rehabilitation Services at Beulahland Natural Medicine Clinic in Thebes Park, Illinois. "A lack of calcium, potassium, and magnesium can make the large muscles in the legs hyperirritable," he says.

Calcium, magnesium, and potassium all have an effect on muscle contraction and relaxation. In addition, they help nerve transmission.

Experts say that you can help calm your legs and get some rest by making sure you get enough of all three minerals. Dr. Hauser recommends taking a daily dose of between 800 and 1,000 milligrams of calcium, 300 milligrams of potassium, and 500 milligrams of magnesium at bedtime.

Try 5-HTP for a good night's sleep. The little jerking movements you make just as you're shifting into sleep are outward signs that your brain is closing the gate on muscle movement for the night. If those muscles didn't voluntarily shut down, they'd go on obeying your brain impulses even in the midst of deep sleep. Without that safety switch, if you dreamed of running a marathon, you might end up about 26 miles from where you went to sleep.

For people with restless legs syndrome, that gating mechanism may not be functioning at 100 percent efficiency, says Dr. Lombard. Some movement impulses are getting through, keeping your legs active all night long and leaving you exhausted come morning.

"The supplement 5-hydroxytryptophan (5-HTP) seems to work well," says Dr. Lombard. Experts believe that 5-HTP is used to make serotonin, a chemical messenger in the brain that can affect sleep quality.

Some people with restless legs who try 5-HTP notice a change for the better right away, but you might have to take the supplements for 2 weeks to a month before you'll know whether it will work for you, according to Dr. Lombard.

Start by taking 100 milligrams about 20 minutes before you go to bed, he suggests. You can increase the dose to 200 milligrams if you don't see results after the first few weeks, but don't take any more than that, he advises. Larger doses can cause disturbing dreams and nightmares.

You shouldn't take 5-HTP for longer than 3 months without consulting a doctor. You should also avoid it if you are currently taking antidepressants or have taken them recently. The combined effects could cause a possibly fatal condition called serotonin syndrome. Do not take supplements of 5-HTP if you are pregnant or trying to conceive.

Stabilize membranes with horse chestnut. Preparations of horse chestnut leaves, bark, and seeds are used in Europe for their good effect on vein health. There's reason to consider standardized extracts of this herb for the treatment of restless legs as well, according to Dr. Hauser.

Give this herbal remedy a try by taking 400 milligrams of standardized extract twice a day, says Dr. Hauser. Generally, people respond within a month, he adds. If your symptoms don't improve in that amount of time, stop taking it and see your doctor for an evaluation.

Horse chestnut is not for everyone. It may interfere with the action of other drugs, especially blood thinners such as warfarin (Coumadin). It may also irritate the gastrointestinal tract. As with other herbs, you should not take it if you are pregnant or breastfeeding.

"You must obtain a standardized extract and follow package directions if you're going to use horse chestnut as a healing herb," says James A. Duke, Ph.D., botanical consultant, former ethnobotanist with the U.S. Department of Agriculture who specializes in medicinal plants, and author of *The Green Pharmacy*. "It's simply not safe to use otherwise."

Sinus Problems

When you take a deep breath, you may inhale hundreds of irritants that can result in clogged sinuses. Among them are pollen, cigarette smoke, dust, cold germs, and exhaust fumes from cars, trucks, buses, and lawn mowers.

And when sinuses are clogged, the mucus they produce often can't drain properly. Fluid builds up, causing pressure and pain—along with any number of problems, from bad breath and stuffy nose to toothache and infection. The natural remedies here—used in conjunction with medical care and with your doctor's approval—may help ease sinus pain, according to some health professionals.

Try garlic. The following remedy for severe and painful bouts of sinus congestion isn't pleasant, but it works fast, says Vasant Lad, B.A.M.S., M.A.Sc., director of the Ayurvedic Institute in Albuquerque, New Mexico.

"Use a garlic press to squeeze fresh garlic juice, then put the juice into an eyedropper," he says. "Put a few drops into your nostrils and keep your head back so that the juice stays inside your nose for about 5 minutes." Then, says Dr.

Lad, sit up and let the garlic juice drain out onto a hand-kerchief or a tissue. He says your sinuses should be quite clear. Use this remedy no more than once a day when needed for sinus congestion, according to Dr. Lad. During a severe sinus attack, he says, it may be repeated up to three times a day—morning, afternoon, and evening.

Turn to the saltwater solution. For less severe sinus problems, a lukewarm saltwater solution may help restore easy breathing, according to Dr. Lad. To make the solution, mix ½ teaspoon of salt in ½ cup of warm water. Then, he says, hold the salt water in the palm of your hand and sniff a bit into each nostril to help drain the sinuses. He suggests using this remedy as needed, up to three times an hour, to clear sinuses.

Take ginger. You can also sniff a pinch of ginger powder into the nostrils to help relieve the pain of swollen sinuses, says David Frawley, O.M.D., director of the American Institute of Vedic Studies in Santa Fe, New Mexico. He says to do this whenever you have sinus congestion. Do not use this remedy if you develop or are prone to bloody noses, he cautions.

When to See a Doctor

- Your sinus pain doesn't improve after taking over-the-counter medication for 3 to 5 days.
- You also have a fever, cough, or headache that has lasted longer than 1 day.
- You develop swollen eyelids and swelling along the sides of your nose.
- You have green or yellowish discharge.
- You have blurred or double vision.

Moisturize your sinuses. To prevent sinus problems from developing, Dr. Lad recommends keeping your nostrils moisturized. "Using an eyedropper, put five drops of warm clarified butter or sesame oil in each nostril," he says. "Do this at least once a day, either in the morning or evening to moisturize your sinuses."

Sesame oil is available in health food stores. To make clarified butter, melt unsalted butter in a heavy saucepan over medium heat. As soon as it begins to boil and foam, reduce the heat to a simmer and cook until golden in color and no foam remains on top. Stir occasionally after the whitish curds sink to the bottom and continue until the curds turn light tan. Cool and strain into a sterile jar. Discard the curds from the bottom. Store tightly sealed at room temperature.

Let food heal you. Barley green, which can be used in juices or simply sprinkled on salads as a topping, helps some people with sinus problems, says Julian Whitaker, M.D., founder and president of the Whitaker Wellness Center in Newport Beach, California. Barley green is available in health food stores.

Hit the hot water bottle. A hot water bottle is a simple, effective way to relieve sinus pain, says Agatha Thrash, M.D., a medical pathologist and cofounder and codirector of Uchee Pines Institute, a natural healing center in Seale, Alabama. Fill about half of the bottle with hot (never boiling) water, wrap it in a towel, and hold it against your nose and forehead until the pain subsides.

Turn on the juice. Both apple and dark grape juices may be beneficial to those with sinus problems, says John Peterson, M.D., an Ayurvedic practitioner in Muncie, Indiana. He recommends drinking the juice at room temperature and apart from meals. You can dilute either juice with water if it seems too strong, he adds.

Use therapeutic vitamins. According to David Edelberg, M.D., an internist and medical director of the American Holistic Center/Chicago, a person with sinus problems may want to try the following regimen of dietary supplements to help relieve symptoms: 2,000 milligrams of vitamin C twice a day; 400 international units of vitamin E twice a day; and 500 milligrams of n-acetylcysteine (available in health food stores) twice a day.

Wash problems away. You can help both prevent and treat sinus problems if you do a yoga nasal wash once a day, says Stephen A. Nezezon, M.D., yoga teacher and staff physician at the Himalayan International Institute of Yoga Science and Philosophy in Honesdale, Pennsylvania. Start by filling a 4-ounce paper cup halfway with warm water, then add ½ teaspoon of salt. Put a small crease in the lip of the cup so that it forms a spout. Slightly tilt your head back and to the left. Then slowly pour the water into your right nostril. The water will flow out of your left nostril or down the back of your throat if your left nostril is clogged. Spit out the water if it goes down your throat; wipe the water from your face with a hand towel if it flows out of your left nostril. Fill the cup again, then repeat the procedure on the other side, pouring the water into your left nostril and tilting your head to the right so that the water flows out of your right nostril.

Skin Itching

Itchy skin is a torment. And the obvious solution—scratching—seems to make things even more itchy. It's not your imagination. Scratching one itch excites other nerves nearby, causing them to itch as well, says Dr. Mitchell C. Stickler of Lewes, Delaware.

What makes us itch in the first place? Usually, it's dry skin, particularly in the cold months. Cold air contains less water vapor than warm air. Heaters remove additional moisture from the air, making the skin even drier, says Dr. Stickler. In winter, the skin loses more moisture to this dry air, causing dry, itchy skin.

Other itch-makers include rashes, insect bites, stress, and even internal diseases, such as cancer.

First of all, don't scratch. It's not good for your skin. "In fact, if you concentrate on scratching a small area of your skin religiously for 5 minutes a day, at the end of the month you would have a nice little thickened area of skin called localized neurodermatitis," says Dr. K. William Kitzmiller of the University of Cincinnati.

Since it's so hard not to scratch, however, it's best to eliminate the itch. Here's how.

Ice the itch. Putting a cold compress on an itchy spot such as a mosquito bite will slow nerve signals so that the area won't feel as itchy, says Dr. Kitzmiller.

Get some fatty acids. Since your body doesn't manufacture essential fatty acids, you have to get them from your diet in foods such as cold-water fish and flaxseed. Or you can take a fatty-acid supplement, available at health food stores. These acids help lubricate your eyes, skin, and throat, says Robert Abel Jr., M.D., clinical professor of ophthalmology at Thomas Jefferson University in Philadelphia.

When taking fatty-acid supplements, start with the lowest dosage. Take it for a month and see if it helps. Then increase the dosage if you need to, Dr. Abel advises.

Be cool and dry. When water evaporates from your skin, it leaves you parched. Hot water tends to be particularly drying. So it's a good idea to keep showers and baths short and not too hot—especially in winter when the air is dry, says Dr. Stickler.

Limit the suds. Soap dries the skin, so don't overdo it. Use it mainly to wash your face, armpits, genitals, and feet, Dr. Stickler says. And use a mild soap such as Oil of Olay, Dove, or Basis or a soapless cleanser like Cetaphil lotion.

Be slippery when wet. Applying a moisturizer while your skin is still wet will help lock in moisture. Smooth it over your entire body, not just your face and hands. "Your legs need more cold-weather moisturizing because they have fewer sebaceous glands to lubricate them naturally," says Amy E. Newburger, M.D., assistant clinical professor of dermatology at Columbia University School of Medicine in New York City.

You don't have to spend a lot of money on a moisturizer. They all do pretty much the same thing, Dr. Stickler says.

Slow Healing

If it seems as if your latest injury is taking a long time to heal, don't despair. With a few changes in diet and lifestyle, you can strengthen your healing forces and speed your recovery.

It's true, however, that your body's wounds are slower to heal as you get older. "That's why it's so important to take good care of yourself as you age, especially with regard to nutrition and activity levels," says Larry Millikan, M.D., chairman of the department of dermatology at Tulane University School of Medicine in New Orleans.

Once you have adequately cleaned and cared for a wound or injury, there are several things you can do to speed healing and recovery. If you're looking for a good place to begin boosting your wound-healing power, start with the dining room table.

Heal with your meals. Even though you may not be as active or have as much appetite as you used to, your body still needs a regular supply of nutritious foods if it's going to be able to stay healthy and make speedy repairs. "Some

When to See a Doctor

- A simple cut takes longer than a week to heal.
- The cut becomes red and swollen.

people eat only one meal a day. Let's say it's dinner, but they've skipped breakfast and had a candy bar for lunch. That's going to weaken their immune systems and slow down their healing," says Dr. Millikan. Try instead to eat three nutritious meals a day.

Put in the protein. Your body requires about 45 grams of protein a day to repair damaged tissues. A 3-ounce serving (about the size of a deck of cards) of fish, chicken, or turkey or cheese will provide about 21 grams of protein. A cup of milk will give you 8 grams of protein, and a half-cup of beans will provide about 7 grams.

Boost immunity with antioxidants. Vitamins C and E as well as beta-carotene (a vitamin A precursor) are all antioxidants, which means they're particularly beneficial in boosting your immune system, helping to fight infection, and promoting more rapid healing, says Frederic Haberman, M.D., assistant clinical professor of medicine (dermatology) at Albert Einstein College of Medicine in New York City and director of the Haberman Dermatology Institute in Ridgewood, New Jersey.

"I tell people to take 500 to 1,000 milligrams of vitamin C, about 400 international units (IU) of E, and up to 2,000 IU of vitamin A after surgery," Dr. Haberman says. "They should also take about 70 micrograms of selenium." Although vitamin E is generally sold in doses of 400 IU, one small study showed a possible risk of stroke in dosages higher than 200 IU. Consult with your doctor if you are at high risk for stroke.

Be zealous about zinc. When it comes to wounds, the mineral zinc has strong healing power, according to Eleanor Young, R.D., Ph.D., a licensed dietitian and professor in the department of medicine at the University of Texas Health Sciences Center in San Antonio.

Dr. Haberman recommends 15 milligrams of zinc per day. You can get it in supplement form, and it's also in foods like steamed oysters and most meat dishes.

Make multis part of a healthy diet. Take a multivitamin and mineral supplement, such as Centrum, says Dr. Millikan.

"The supplement provides the antioxidants and minerals needed to promote a stronger immune response," says Dr. Haberman.

Go for aloe. Buy an aloe plant to keep on the shelf as a houseplant, suggests Dr. Millikan. The next time you cut yourself, break off a leaf, split it lengthwise, and use the juice to speed healing. "Many of my patients firmly believe that this is a great help," he says. Research has shown that aloe can penetrate and numb tissue, reduce swelling, improve blood flow, and prevent the growth of harmful bacteria, fungi, and virus.

Walk your wounds off. People who exercise regularly tend to heal more rapidly and are more likely to have stronger immune systems. "The key is good blood circulation," says Dr. Millikan. As long as your tissues get enough blood, they're also getting adequate oxygen, nutrients, and immune cells—all the ingredients they need in order to heal. "On the other hand, people who have circulatory disorders tend to heal more slowly and can suffer from more infections," Dr. Millikan observes. One circulation problem that can slow healing is atherosclerosis, or hardening of the arteries, a condition that impedes blood flow. Another is diabetes—the inability to incorporate blood sugar, which leaves body cells deprived of nutrition and wounds more susceptible to infection.

For most people, the best exercise is walking, says Dr. Millikan. "You shouldn't adopt an exercise program, even walking, without first consulting your doctor to see how much exercise you can do safely. Once your doctor gives you the okay, walking is an ideal way to promote circulation and more rapid healing."

Snoring

Excess neck fat is a major cause of snoring. The fat chokes off room for air to travel. Then, when you lie down at night, gravity pulls tissues in the mouth and throat downward, choking off still more room. With each breath, that hanging tissue vibrates. And your bed partner hears "Hhgzzzzz."

Though fat is a common cause of snoring, anything that narrows airways in the nose, mouth, or throat—like an overbite, stuffy nose, or enlarged tonsils—can have the same effect.

Snoring is more than merely a nuisance to your bed-mate. Over time, it can strain the heart, contributing to heart disease. Snorers also tend to develop high blood pressure at a younger age than nonsnorers.

In some cases, home remedies like the following are all that you'll need to silence a snore. But if you suspect that you have the more serious condition sleep apnea (during which breathing stops for short periods of time), do yourself a favor and see your doctor.

Prop up your bed. Placing bricks or blocks of wood under the two legs at the head of your bed will elevate your upper body slightly. This will reduce gravity's effect on your tongue and help to keep airways open, advises Edmund Pribitkin, M.D., an otolaryngologist at Thomas Jefferson University Hospital in Philadelphia.

Avoid alcohol, tranquilizers, and antihistamines before bedtime. Each of these has effects that can make your muscles overly relaxed and contribute to snoring, says Alex Clerk, M.D., director of the sleep disorders clinic at Stanford University.

Try decongestants or steroid nasal sprays. They combat nasal congestion that might be contributing to snoring, Dr. Clerk says.

Stay off your back. Sleeping on your back allows the tongue to fall backward into your throat, narrowing the airway. Some experts advise sewing a small pouch in the back of a T-shirt or pajama top and putting a tennis ball inside. The resulting bulge will help you resist the urge to roll over onto your back at night, even when you're asleep.

Whistle while you work. Research suggests that singing and whistling may help to tone the very muscles that want to fall forward when you sleep. By incorporating singing or whistling into your daily routine, you may help cut down on the cacophony at night.

Skip the snack. Avoid nibbling 3 hours before retiring. The process of digestion causes muscles everywhere—including those in your throat—to loosen up.

Shed some pounds. People who snore and have sleep apnea tend to have a neck circumference of 17 inches or more—about the size of a supermodel's waist. Trimming down can cure snoring and sleep apnea in some people. At the very least, it can play an important role in any stop-snoring plan. "It's a good recommendation to lose weight because it will help make other treatments more effective," says Dr. Clerk.

Stop being a butt head. Studies show that smoking can

aggravate snoring. The best thing you can do is quit entirely, but even cutting back may help.

Wear a retainer. A specially trained dentist or orthodontist can fit you with an oral appliance that will keep your tongue from falling backward into your throat, which can help reduce snoring, says John Ruddy, M.D., assistant clinical professor at the National Jewish Center/University of Colorado Health Sciences Center in Denver.

Use a mask. Wearing a pressurized mask when you sleep is perhaps the most effective way to treat snoring, says Dr. Clerk. This system, called continuous positive airway pressure (CPAP), maintains the upper airway in an open position while you sleep.

The drawback is that wearing a mask at night can be cumbersome, inconvenient, and even claustrophobic. It's a good idea to try as many different masks and machines as you can, since some are more comfortable than others, says Dr. Ruddy.

Consider surgery. For mild to moderate snoring problems, surgical treatment has come a long way, says Jack Coleman, M.D., of Nashville, chairman of the sleep disorders committee for the American Academy of Otolaryngology–Head and Neck Surgery. Today, a doctor can use a laser to vaporize excess tissue, which in some cases can eliminate snoring altogether. It's a simple outpatient procedure that's done with a local anesthetic. Some people, however, need multiple sessions over a 6-month period, says Dr. Coleman.

Sore Throat

The raw, burning sensation of a sore throat is an extremely common symptom that usually means you have an inflammation somewhere between the back of your tongue and your voice box.

Often it is the first sign of a cold, the flu, or a viral or bacterial infection such as strep throat or mononucleosis. In other cases, that tickle in your throat can be caused by dry indoor air, allergies, or exposure to smoke, chemicals, or pollution. In most cases, a sore throat will subside on its own in a few days. The natural remedies here may also help.

Smell good. To speed the healing of a sore throat, Los Angeles aromatic consultant John Steele recommends applying a thin film of canola, sunflower, grape seed, or safflower oil externally on your neck over the throat area. Apply seven drops of sandalwood essential oil over the oil and rub gently into the skin, suggests Steele. "This treatment is soothing and smells wonderful," he explains. Or, he says, add two drops of tea tree, ginger, sandalwood, or geranium essential oil to ½ ounce of warm water and gargle. Any of these essential oils can be taken with a spoonful of honey to coat the throat, says Steele. Essential oils are available in health food stores.

Gargle with turmeric. Stir ½ teaspoon of salt and 1 teaspoon of turmeric into a cup of hot water and gargle with this mixture before going to bed, says Vasant Lad, B.A.M.S., M.A.Sc., director of the Ayurvedic Institute in Albuquerque, New Mexico. If your sore throat doesn't go away within a few days, see a doctor, he adds.

Let garlic help. Allicin, the compound that puts the pungent odor in garlic, has antibiotic and antifungal properties that can heal many types of sore throat, says registered pharmacist Earl Mindell, R.Ph., Ph.D., professor of nutrition at Pacific Western University in Los Angeles and author of *Earl Mindell's Food as Medicine* and other books on nutrition. Take two or more cloves, crushed or whole, at the first sign of a sore throat and continue eating two cloves a day until your symptoms clear up, he says.

Raw garlic is the most effective, says Dr. Mindell, but it can cause gastrointestinal upset. He suggests baking and stir-frying as other ways of getting garlic into your diet. Or, he says, take garlic supplements for all of the benefits with none of the digestive upset. Garlic supplements are available in health food stores; Dr. Mindell recommends taking three capsules twice a day with meals until your symptoms clear up.

Turn to herbs. Try gargling with goldenseal tea, says Varro E. Tyler, Ph.D., professor of pharmacognosy at Purdue University in West Lafayette, Indiana. To make the tea, Dr. Tyler says to pour boiling water over 1 to 2 teaspoons of the dried herb, which you can buy in health food stores. Steep for 10 minutes, strain to remove the herb, and cool before using as a mouthwash, he says.

Sage is another good choice for a sore throat, according to Dr. Tyler. He says to chop 2 teaspoons of fresh leaves, then pour boiling water over them and steep for 10 minutes. Strain the tea to remove the leaves and cool before using as a mouthwash, he says. Dr. Tyler suggests that you repeat the gargles as necessary for a maximum of 2 to 3 days.

Suck on an unusual lozenge. "Charcoal has been shown to adhere to certain pathogenic germs that cause sore throats," says Agatha Thrash, M.D., a medical pathologist and cofounder and codirector of Uchee Pines Institute, a natural healing center in Seale, Alabama. Using activated charcoal powder (available in health food stores and some drugstores) and cold water, make a paste thick enough to roll into a ball. Suck on the ball as long as it lasts to heal a sore throat fast, suggests Dr. Thrash.

Heal with juice. Ginger and pineapple both contain natural anti-inflammatory agents that can speed the

When to See a Doctor

- The pain lasts for more than 2 to 3 days.
- You also have a fever of 101°F or higher, difficulty swallowing, swollen glands in your neck, or white patches on your tonsils or in the area where your tonsils used to be.
- You also have a reddish, sandpaper-like rash on your trunk.
- You have a history of rheumatic fever.
- You have been exposed to either strep throat or mononucleosis or there is a community outbreak.
- You get sore throats frequently but haven't been to the doctor.

healing of a sore throat, according to Cherie Calbom, M.S., a certified nutritionist in Kirkland, Washington, and co-author of *Juicing for Life*. She suggests juicing three pineapple rings together with a ¼-inch-thick slice of fresh ginger for a delicious healing cocktail.

Sip hot lemonade. It's not lemonade in the traditional sense, but it can ease the pain of a sore throat. Combine half lemon juice and half tea; add enough honey to sweeten it then coat your throat. "It makes your throat feel good," says Penelope Shar, M.D., an internist in private practice in Bangor, Maine.

Load up on vitamin C. Whether caused by a virus, pollutants, or just misusing your voice, a sore throat usually means that a more acute infection will follow. Vitamin C can help prevent infection and speed up the healing process, says Richard Gerson, Ph.D., author of *The Right Vitamins*. He says you can safely take up to 10,000 milligrams a day of vitamin C at the first sign of a problem, provided you drink plenty of water to flush away excess amounts of the nutrient.

Stomach Pain

Medically speaking, there's no such thing as a stomachache. That's because what we think of as a stomachache could really be any of a number of abdomen-related pains—a dull ache, bloating, sharp cramps, acid pain, gas pain, or even pain related to diarrhea or constipation.

The possible causes are just as diverse: stress, dyspepsia (more commonly called indigestion), heartburn, gallstones, ulcers, lactose intolerance, or irritable bowel syndrome. You might be overeating or not eating enough. You might have eaten food that was ill-prepared, spoiled, or that simply didn't agree with you.

This much is certain: As you age, your digestive system may become more particular about what it can and can't handle, says Martin Brotman, M.D., gastroenterologist at the California Pacific Medical Center in San Francisco. And when your system has to deal with something it doesn't like, it will probably let you know about it—often in the form of a stomachache. But if you're armed with that knowledge, you can soothe or prevent most stomachaches, no matter what's causing them, with some simple strategies.

Go through the process of elimination. Since your digestive processes get more finicky every year, that increases the likelihood that a certain food, beverage, or medication can cause a stomachache. "Try eliminating different things, such as aspirin, to see if you feel better," says Dr. Brotman.

Even chewing gum should come under suspicion. Some people get abdominal cramps and diarrhea when they chew sugar-free gum that's made with the sweetener sorbitol. Dairy foods and beverages such as ice cream and milk are other common offenders that can make you feel more gassy and bloated, as are many high-sugar or high-fat foods. If you suspect that a food is causing the problem, take it out of your diet for a few days. If the stomachache disappears, you've found your culprit, says Dr. Brotman.

Give your belly a break. You can help your stomach recover from a bellyache by going on just liquids for the rest of the day, says Dr. Brotman. Stick to clear liquids, such as chicken broth, flat ginger ale, and water. Avoid carbonated or caffeinated beverages.

Loosen up. If you have a bloated, sore belly, make yourself more comfortable by wearing loose clothing. Loosen your belt. If you're wearing a tight skirt or pants, change into trousers, sweats, or pajama bottoms that have a bigger waistband, until your stomach settles down.

Warm your tummy. Turn a heating pad on low and place it on your abdomen until the pain subsides, says Dr. Brotman. "Warmth on the abdomen offers some comfort. If the pain continues for several hours and is new to you, notify your doctor."

Take time out. Soothe a sore stomach with rest. Put up your feet. Relax. "Close your eyes," suggests Roger L. Gebhard, M.D., gastroenterologist at the Veterans Affairs Medical Center and professor of medicine in the division of gastroenterology at the University of Minnesota, both in Minneapolis. "Find in your memory a place you've been

When to See a Doctor

- Your stomachache is so severe that you're doubled over.
- It is accompanied by nausea and vomiting that lasts longer than 1 to 2 days or keeps coming back.
- The ache is accompanied by a change in bowel habits (constipation or diarrhea) and is accompanied by fever or blood in your stool.

to. A place of beauty, maybe a lake or a campground or a beach. Go back to that spot in your mind. Sit on a rock. Listen to the natural sounds. Breathe naturally."

Welcome a little BRAT into your home. When you are ready to eat a little something, try the BRAT diet—bananas, rice, applesauce, or toast. These foods are all easy for your stomach to digest. "Don't rush back into solid food by eating a steak dinner," says Dr. Brotman.

Call on chamomile. Chamomile tea is an age-old and, many believe, effective herbal remedy to ease a sore belly, says Mike Cantwell, M.D., clinician and coordinator for clinical research at the Institute for Health and Healing at the California Pacific Medical Center. Try two or three 6-ounce cups a day, between meals. Chamomile decreases stomach activity and helps coat the stomach as well, says Dr. Cantwell. You can find the tea in most grocery stores. Follow the directions on tea-bag packages. If you are using loose dried chamomile flowers, steep 1 teaspoon of chamomile in boiling water for 10 to 15 minutes. Very rarely, chamomile can cause an allergic reaction when ingested. People who are allergic to closely related plants such as ragweed, asters, and chrysanthemums should drink the tea with caution.

Stay regular. Constipation can certainly lead to stomach distress, so make sure that you're getting a healthy dose of fiber every day. Shoot for 25 grams, says Dr. Gebhard. Include apples, bran, cabbage, and raw vegetables in your diet—and drink eight 8-ounce glasses of water a day to help keep you regular. "Peel the apple if the skin is hard for you to chew or digest," adds Dr. Gebhard.

Don't overfill with fiber. Believe it or not, stomach problems can also be caused by too much of a good thing—specifically, fiber. For some people, eating more fiber than they are accustomed to can cause gas and abdominal bloating, says Dr. Gebhard. It's best to introduce fiber into your diet slowly and a little at a time. Dr. Gebhard recommends starting with 10 to 15 grams a day, increasing by 5 grams each week to 25.

Work out stress. Tension and stress can cause plenty of stomach pain. To help relieve stress, put some regular exercise into your weekly routine. Try walking for a half-hour 3 days a week, says Wanda Filer, M.D., a family-practice physician in York, Pennsylvania. When you're active, you'll also find that your bowel movements become more regular, which is helpful if constipation is causing your abdominal distress.

Eat mindfully. That means paying attention to the role of food in your daily life, says Amy Saltzman, M.D., internist for the Institute for Health and Healing at the California Pacific Medical Center.

"By bringing attention to when, what, where, and how you eat, you may improve not only your digestion but also the quality of your life," says Dr. Saltzman. "Try eating a mindful meal. Prepare the food with attention to what will be satisfying—and eat when you are hungry." When you sit down to eat, be sure to go slowly, Dr. Saltzman adds. Concentrate on eating and taste each bite before you swallow.

Stress

Daily traffic. Work deadlines. Family squabbles. Rebellious teenagers. Illness. Injury. All of these life experiences add up to big-time stress that can knock you off your feet, spin you around, and keep you dazed. Without some relief, you may feel as if each morning is the beginning of a new melodrama.

Poking fun at stress is one way to help you de-stress. But the truth is stress is no laughing matter. Whenever you're filled with tension and anxiety, your adrenal glands, located above your kidneys, pump out stress hormones such as adrenaline and cortisol, which give your body that burst of energy it needs to escape danger. Long-term stress causes chronically high levels of stress hormones, which can weaken your immune system, tax your heart and blood vessels, tire you out, and make you more susceptible to illness.

Fortunately, certain dietary and lifestyle changes can help relieve stress and release tension.

Get moving. For starters, get at least 20 minutes of aerobic exercise three to five times a week to lift your spirits and melt away feelings of pressure and anxiety. Also, don't overlook weight lifting and brisk walking, as they can have similar effects.

Set limits. Another tip for stress control: Limit your intake of caffeine, alcohol, high-fat foods, and sugar. Caffeine and alcohol can raise the levels of stress hormones in the blood and alter brain chemistry. Caffeine also causes nervousness, anxiety, and irritability. Moreover, when you replace nutritious foods with refined carbohydrates like sugar, you lower the amount of vitamins and minerals in your diet, depleting your body of essential nutrients that protect you from the dangers of stress.

Take C and see what happens. Vitamin C gives your immune system the fighting power it needs to prevent many stress-related health problems such as headaches, high blood pressure, diabetes, and heart disease, says C. Norman Shealy, M.D., Ph.D., founder of the American Holistic Medical Association and director of the Shealy Institute, an alternative medicine clinic in Springfield, Missouri.

What's more, vitamin C is required to manufacture stress hormones, which can flow excessively if you're stressed for a long time. After a while, your adrenal glands become exhausted from overwork, and your body's ability to produce stress hormones declines, says Ray Sahelian, M.D., a physician in Marina del Rey, California, and author of *Kava: The Miracle Antianxiety Herb*. Once this happens, you could experience excessive fatigue, low blood pressure, and low blood sugar. Supplementing with extra vitamin C is one step that you can take to keep your adrenal glands healthy.

When the going gets tough, take 3,000 milligrams of vitamin C in divided doses daily, says Dr. Shealy.

Welcome the B family. The B-complex vitamins are a treasure trove of stress relief. They can give you more energy, strip away fatigue, make adrenal gland hormones, and manufacture brain chemicals responsible for keeping you alert and lifting your mood, says Dr. Sahelian. "The B vitamins work in concert with each other, and they play hundreds of biochemical roles in the body," he says.

Feed Your Adrenal Glands

To zap fatigue, boost energy, and cope with stress, some people turn to adrenal gland extracts. Advocates claim these products can put life back into your own adrenal glands, which have become tired out from long periods of stress. Doctors know that without healthy adrenal glands, we're more prone to infections and stress-related illnesses.

The results aren't certain, however. "It's believed that adrenal extracts can help people who are under a great deal of stress or who have chronic fatigue, but very little research has been done to prove their effectiveness, and dosages aren't standardized," says C. Norman Shealy, M.D., Ph.D., founder of the American Holistic Medical Association. He notes that some people could benefit, however.

To find the right dosage, you may need to experiment, according to Joseph E. Pizzorno Jr., N.D., president of Bastyr University in Bothell, Washington. "I suggest taking one-third the recommended dosage on the label and slowly increasing it every 2 days unless you notice any signs of irritability, restlessness, or insomnia. If you experience any of these symptoms, simply reduce your dosage until they go away. Over time, you should notice an increase in energy and better resistance to stress." If you don't feel better in 2 to 3 weeks, the supplements are probably not working for you.

The members of this close-knit family include thiamin, riboflavin, niacin, pantothenic acid, and vitamins B_6 and B_{12}. Pantothenic acid, in particular, plays a major role in the making of adrenal gland hormones and energy production, says Dr. Sahelian.

If you want to combat stress, check with a doctor or naturopath about taking a daily high-potency B-complex vitamin formula that includes 100 to 500 milligrams of pantothenic acid, 50 to 75 milligrams of vitamin B_6, and 500 micrograms of B_{12}, says Joseph E. Pizzorno Jr., N.D., president of Bastyr University in Bothell, Washington.

Try a stress-busting powerhouse. Ginseng is considered the most notable medicinal herb used to restore vitality, boost energy, reduce fatigue, improve mental and physical performance, and protect the body from the negative effects of stress. With ginseng, your initial reaction to stress is likely to be less intense. It's often referred to as a tonic for the adrenal glands because it tones and maintains their overall health.

You can find different varieties of the herb. Asian ginseng is the most widely used for medicinal purposes and is more of a stimulant than its Siberian cousin, says Dr. Pizzorno. Thus, if you're acutely stressed or recovering from a long illness, Asian ginseng would be the way to go.

Because potency varies, as does the concentration of active ingredients, you'll need to adjust the amount you take depending on which product you buy. You can take 1,000 to 2,000 milligrams one to three times a day if you choose a high-quality crude Asian ginseng root, says Dr. Pizzorno. If you take an extract standardized to 5 to 7 percent ginsenosides, take 100 milligrams one to three times a day.

If you're taking Siberian ginseng root, says Dr. Pizzorno, you probably should take somewhere between 2,000 and 3,000 milligrams a day in divided doses. If you take the extract, take 100 to 200 milligrams of a product that is standardized to 0.8 percent eleutherosides three times a day. Because everyone's response to ginseng is different, start off with the lower dosage and increase it over time, he suggests.

Women taking Asian ginseng may experience breast tenderness. You can simply reduce the dose or discontinue use to make the symptoms go away, says Dr. Pizzorno.

Cool out with kava kava. This time-honored herb can calm your nerves and help you unwind. Not only that, it's fast-acting, so you may see the effects in as little as 30 to 60 minutes.

Kava can actually preempt stress if you take it prior to an expected stressful situation. It's also a post-stress soother: You can take it to relax tense muscles and wind yourself down after an especially stressful day. You'll feel at peace and maybe even a little euphoric, says Dr. Sahelian. The secret behind kava is its anxiety-reducing effect on your brain.

What's more, kava isn't addictive, it won't lose its effectiveness over time, and your mind will remain alert and sharp even when you take it during the day.

Dr. Sahelian suggests taking one capsule that contains between 40 and 70 milligrams of kavalactones two or three times a day. Start with the lower dosage first to determine whether you feel any of the soothing effects, he says. If you don't feel any stress relief in 2 to 3 hours, you can take another capsule.

Taste Loss

If you don't smell things as well as you once did, there could be many explanations. Advancing age can be a contributing factor, possibly because infection has taken its toll or because you've sniffed too many noxious fumes over the years. Moreover, you shouldn't be surprised if you temporarily lose your sense of smell because you've had an infection such as a bad cold.

Head injury is another possible cause if the delicate nerves leading from your nose to your brain are damaged. Also, certain prescription drugs can rob you of some ability to enjoy the fragrance of flowers, perfume, or fresh-baked apple pie.

As smell slips away, your sense of taste may suffer, too. The two senses are so closely related that people who complain of not being able to smell often say that they also have trouble tasting.

Depending on the cause, disturbances of taste and smell can be permanent. Yet you also might regain these senses after a while, says Charles P. Kimmelman, M.D., associate professor of otolaryngology at Weill Medical

College of Cornell University in New York City and attending physician at Manhattan Eye, Ear, and Throat Hospital. If smell loss is linked to a head cold, for instance, you can expect your nose to work normally after you've shaken off the cold.

When the problems last longer, talk to your doctor. "Disturbances of the taste and smell senses are best treated by a physician," says Barbara Silbert, D.C., N.D., a chiropractor and naturopathic doctor in Newburyport, Massachusetts. Meanwhile, here are other things you can try.

Develop a taste for heavy metal. The cells in your taste buds and nose that help you to smell depend on zinc. In fact, cells in the salivary glands make a zinc-dependent protein called gustin that is secreted into your saliva. An important contributor to your sense of taste, gustin helps develop cells that can distinguish among different flavors.

Although long-term zinc deficiencies are pretty rare in the United States, it's worth asking your doctor to test for a deficiency if you are experiencing taste and smell loss. Many things can lead to a deficiency, including poor eating habits, alcoholism, certain drugs, kidney disease, and the stress of surgery or serious burns.

"If I discover a zinc deficiency, I typically recommend 25 milligrams of zinc picolinate twice a day to start," says Dr. Silbert. Of course, you can also eat more of the foods that contain zinc. Your best bet is seafood such as cooked oysters and crab. Meats such as lean beef and lean pork also provide zinc, but they're also high in saturated fat. Other sources include eggs, whole grains, nuts, and yogurt. If you plan to take more than 20 milligrams of zinc a day, it's best to do so under your doctor's care.

Toothache

A toothache is usually an early sign of a cavity. But it also can be caused by inflammation of the gums, an abscess (an infection that develops in the tooth root or between the tooth and gum), a cracked tooth, or a dislodged filling. Each of these problems can cause different types of toothache, says Flora Parsa Stay, D.D.S., a dentist in Oxnard, California, and author of *The Complete Book of Dental Remedies*. Your dentist will probably suspect that you have a cracked tooth, for instance, if you have pressure and pain while chewing. Severe pain accompanied by sensitivity to hot and cold could be a sign that a cavity has reached the nerve of the tooth.

The following remedies can help soothe your tooth pain while you're waiting for an appointment with your dentist.

String it up. Sometimes, a toothache is caused by something as simple as trapped food between the teeth. These food particles actually irritate the gums, but the pain can radiate into the surrounding teeth, Dr. Stay says. So try rinsing your mouth with warm water to loosen any food particles. Then floss or use a water-irrigating device to clean between your teeth. But even if this technique relieves your pain, you should still consult a dentist to make sure other more complex dental problems aren't contributing to your toothache, she says.

Gnaw a knot of cloves. Take a couple of cloves from a spice rack and place them between your aching tooth and your cheek—much like you'd use chewing tobacco. They can help soothe the pain, says Richard D. Fischer, D.D.S., a dentist in Annandale, Virginia, and past president of the International Academy of Oral Medicine and Toxicology. Let the hard seedlike cloves soak in your mouth's saliva for several minutes to soften them up. Then gently chew on them—like you would on a toothpick—so the soothing oils within the cloves are released into the area surrounding your aching tooth. Leave the cloves in place for about 30 minutes or until the pain subsides. Continue this treatment as needed until you can see a dentist, he suggests.

Lay on the ointment. If gnashing on cloves is unappetizing, then consider using an over-the-counter tooth-pain ointment such as Anbesol or Orajel, Dr. Fischer suggests. Be sure to follow the directions on the label.

Make some waves. Swishing warm salt water around in your mouth can help reduce gum swelling, disinfect abscesses, and relieve tooth pain. Mix a teaspoon of salt into an 8-ounce glass of warm water and use as needed for discomfort, Dr. Fischer says. Swish each mouthful for 10 to 30 seconds, focusing the salt water on the painful area as much as possible. Repeat until the glass is empty. Do this as needed throughout the day, he suggests.

If you have high blood pressure and are on a sodium-restricted diet, use Epsom salt instead of table salt, he says. Epsom salts are made with magnesium and, unlike table salt, shouldn't adversely affect your blood pressure.

Pop a pain reliever. Simply taking a 325-milligram aspirin tablet every 4 to 6 hours can dampen a lot of tooth pain and gum inflammation, says Robert Henry, D.M.D., a dentist in Lexington, Kentucky, and past president of the American Society for Geriatric Dentistry. If you can't tolerate aspirin, then try taking 200 milligrams of ibuprofen every 4 hours, Dr. Henry suggests. Ibuprofen is a potent anti-inflammatory that is gentler on the stomach than aspirin.

If you do use aspirin, never put it directly on the tooth or gums, Dr. Henry urges. Remember, aspirin is an acid. Keeping it in your mouth for more than a few seconds can cause a painful burn that will only complicate the treatment of your toothache.

Try an ice treatment. Wrap an ice pack in a towel and apply it to the outside of your mouth for 15 to 20 minutes every hour until your pain subsides, Dr. Fischer suggests. The ice will reduce swelling and calm agitated nerve endings in your aching tooth.

Load up on minerals. Increasing your intake of calcium and magnesium can help soothe nerves and temporarily ease tooth pain, Dr. Fischer says. He suggests taking 500 milligrams of calcium and 200 to 300 milligrams of magnesium at the first sign of a toothache. *Note:* People with heart or kidney problems should check with their doctors before taking supplemental magnesium.

Invite your teeth to tea. Herbal teas made with chamomile or echinacea often can quell mild toothache pain, Dr. Stay says.

To prepare a chamomile tea, add 2 tablespoons of dried chamomile flowers to 2 cups of boiling water and steep for 10 minutes. As for echinacea, add 4 tablespoons of the dried herb to 8 cups of boiling water and steep for 10 minutes. After they have been strained, you can drink either of these teas as needed for pain, Dr. Stay says. You can also buy these teas premade in the tea section at your health food store. They may not be as strong as the do-it-yourself versions, but they're a little more convenient.

Very rarely, chamomile can cause an allergic reaction when ingested. People allergic to closely related plants such as ragweed, asters, and chrysanthemums should drink the tea with caution. Don't use echinacea if you have autoimmune conditions such as lupus, tuberculosis, or multiple sclerosis. Don't·use it if you're allergic to plants in the daisy family, such as chamomile and marigold.

Picture yourself pain-free. Your imagination is a powerful healer that can help you dampen tooth pain, Dr. Fischer says.

To try it, imagine swimming in ice-cold water or playing in the snow. Feel the chill of the water or snow penetrating your hands and feet so that they are almost numb. Now imagine that feeling of numbness enveloping your aching tooth, soothing it as if you were rubbing it with snow until all of the pain is gone, says Deena Margetis, a certified clinical hypnotherapist specializing in dental care in Annandale, Virginia. Doing this imagery for 1 to 2 minutes as needed may relieve much of your pain, she says.

Urination Problems

Complaints of burning during urination, often accompanied by frequent urges, send eight million women to the doctor's office every year. The usual source of the problem is a urinary tract infection (UTI). One out of every five women gets a urinary tract infection at least once a year, and of those, about 15 percent contract more than three a year.

Women are more prone than men to these infections because both the rectum and the vagina are perfect incubators for bacteria that all too easily find their way into the nearby urethra, the exit tube for urine. And since the female urethra is not very long, it provides an easy route for the bacteria to invade the bladder, causing cystitis. The bacteria can even move farther upstream to the kidneys, causing a more serious infection called pyelonephritis.

A number of other factors can cause or aggravate a burning sensation when you urinate, according to Tamara G. Bavendam, M.D., assistant professor of urology and director of female urology at the University of Washington Medical Center in Seattle. Possible irritants include spicy foods, coffee, tea, alcohol, acidic foods and beverages, chemicals in hygiene products and trauma from sex. Yeast infections can also cause burning.

Depending on the cause, there are two keys to getting rid of that burning sensation: Eliminate the bacteria that cause infections or avoid the irritants. These tips will help.

Flood your bladder. At the first hint of burning, drink two 8-ounce glasses of water, recommends Kristene E. Whitmore, M.D., chief of urology at Graduate Hospital in Philadelphia, clinical associate professor of urology at the University of Pennsylvania, and co-author of *Overcoming Bladder Disorders*. Then dissolve 1 teaspoon baking soda in 4 ounces of water and drink that. Then, for the next 6 to 8 hours, drink 8 ounces of water every hour. Consult your doctor if the symptom is not relieved after a day.

What you're doing is diluting your bacteria-filled urinary tract and forcing yourself to urinate, rather than holding it in, which prolongs the infection. "Oftentimes, the water is enough to flush out the bacteria and make the symptoms tolerable," Dr. Whitmore says. "Sometimes that's all that's needed."

See the doctor. If the burning remains after a day, you should see the doctor. If you're experiencing the burning for the first time, you'll need to give the doctor a urine specimen to check for bacteria. The doctor also will check for a yeast infection or sexually transmitted disease.

Antibiotics in combination with the baking soda and water may rid you of the problem, but if it persists or recurs, more extensive testing will be required, says Dr. Whitmore. That could include more urine cultures, an ultrasound of your kidneys, or running a scope up your urethra for a close-up look at your bladder.

Don't feed the burn. Many foods and drinks can irritate the urinary tract, either causing or aggravating the burning, Dr. Bavendam says. These include alcohol, coffee, tea, chocolate, carbonated beverages, all citrus fruits, tomatoes, chili, spicy foods, vinegar, and sugar. Even decaffeinated coffee can be an irritant, Dr. Whitmore says.

Eliminating all of these foods from your diet can ease the burning and other urinary discomforts within about 10 days, according to Dr. Bavendam. Once the burning sensation is gone, you can start adding them back to your diet one at a time to see which cause a problem. As you do so, she emphasizes, drink a minimum of 1 quart of water throughout the day.

Ease the pain. Urinating through an inflamed urethra or letting urine touch infected or raw skin is like rubbing

Dribble Control

Usually, it's not more than a few drops and isn't a sign of a serious health problem. But it's annoying and leaves little wet spots on your underwear. Fortunately, it is often easy to correct.

Sit back, sit wide. Urinating with your legs wide apart helps prevent any urine from pooling in the vagina or the urethra, from which it can later leak. Leaning forward also helps, says Kevin Pranikoff, M.D., associate professor of urology at the State University of New York at Buffalo.

Give it a squeeze. Kegel exercises can help you strengthen the muscles in the pelvis and gain better control. And they're simple to do. The muscles you want to strengthen are the ones you use to start and stop the flow of urine. Squeeze and slowly release those muscles several times. Urologists recommend that you practice this action until you can contract those muscles 50 times in a row several times a day.

salt into an open wound. To ease that pain, try urinating while sitting in a tub of warm water or while standing in the shower, Dr. Bavendam suggests.

Wipe right. Wipe yourself from front to back after a bowel movement. Doing the reverse can more easily sweep bacteria from your rectum into your urethra.

Practice clean sex. Sex can be a significant source of burning by irritating the urethra or introducing bacteria. "Urinate after having sex," Dr. Bavendam suggests. And after you urinate, says Dr. Whitmore, wash your vagina with a handheld showerhead or bathe it in some water with a tablespoon or so of baking soda.

Stay free of chemicals. Pay particular attention to whether soaps or hygiene products cause irritation, Dr. Bavendam says. Bubble baths, douches, deodorants, and scented toilet papers all contain chemicals that can irritate your urethra or the skin surrounding it.

Dry up. In the summer, don't lounge about in a wet bathing suit, which may stimulate a vaginal yeast or bacteria infection. "Wash off the chlorine," Dr. Whitmore says. "And I tell women to carry a spare bathing suit. Change into the dry one after swimming."

Another problem that affects some people is excessive urination. Assuming you have no underlying medical problems, there is nothing wrong with producing a lot of urine. In fact, "for the health of your bladder, you need to put out about 1 to 2 liters of urine per day," says Margaret M. Baumann, M.D., associate chief of staff for geriatrics and extended care at the Veterans Administration West Side Medical Center in Chicago. If you don't excrete that much, your urine will be too concentrated with wastes, she says. That can harm the lining of the bladder, leading to the formation of kidney stones or causing the bladder to contract even when it's not full.

If you're uncomfortable with your output, though, you might want to try some of these tips.

Measure your output. The first step in taking any action about your urine output is measuring it. To do that, over the course of a 24-hour period, urinate into a soda bottle or jar calibrated for liters or quarts. (Two liters equals a little more than 2 quarts.) If you want a really accurate record, says Dr. Baumann, also note what and when you drink and when you urinate.

Get checked. "If you're producing 6 or more liters of urine a day," says Dr. Baumann, "you might want to get an examination to see if you're diabetic."

Put a muzzle on your guzzle. If you excrete, say, 4 to 5 liters a day, try cutting your liquid intake in half, Dr. Baumann suggests. "You won't be a healthier person by producing more than 1 to 2 liters of urine a day," she says. Besides, while generating a high volume of urine won't necessarily cause incontinence, it may contribute to it, she says.

Don't be a stranger to the restroom. What you perceive as emitting too much urine at one time may be the result of too few trips to the bathroom. If you habitually resist the urge to urinate, you'll enlarge the capacity of your bladder and may also cause a bladder infection, says Joseph M. Montella, M.D., an assistant professor of Obstetrics and Gynecology at Jefferson Medical College of Thomas Jefferson University in Philadelphia. At the worst extreme, your bladder eventually could become so big and so out of shape that it loses its ability to contract.

To maintain a strong bladder that doesn't have an overly expanded capacity, Dr. Montella says, urinate according to a schedule, about every 3 to 4 hours, whether you feel the urge or not.

Vaginal Itching

Vaginitis is an umbrella term for inflammation, irritation, and redness of the vulva and vagina. The most common form is bacterial vaginosis, an infection characterized by a yellowish, fishy-smelling discharge. Yeast infection is another form, which reveals itself with a white, cottage cheese–like discharge, intense itching, and burning.

Trichomoniasis is yet another type, an inflammation triggered by a single-celled organism that's transmitted sexually and causes itching, burning, and a frothy green or yellowish, foul-smelling discharge. Due to hormone level changes, women are more likely to be plagued by vaginitis before menstruation, during pregnancy, or after menopause, when thinning vaginal walls caused by decreasing estrogen become more susceptible to infection. This same lack of estrogen also causes vaginal dryness, which can lead to irritation, inflammation, and a higher risk of developing a bacterial infection.

Whatever the cause or the symptoms, vaginitis needs attention. If left untreated, trichomoniasis can put you at risk for other sexually transmitted diseases, and untreated bacterial vaginosis may lead to urinary tract infections and pelvic inflammatory disease, which can cause infertility. Be sure to see your doctor without delay if you have any of these symptoms.

Here are other things you can do.

Make dietary changes. If you're plagued by chronic yeast infections, some dietary changes could help prevent recurrences. Try to eliminate sugar and milk and other dairy products from your diet, naturopathic doctors advise. You also should avoid foods that contain mold and yeast, including alcoholic beverages, cheeses, dried fruit, melons, mushrooms, and peanuts.

The rationale: *Candida albicans*, the fungus that causes yeast infections, thrives on sugar, and because milk is high in lactose—also a sugar—it may contribute to a yeast infection.

Fight back with vitamin A. This vitamin is a renowned infection fighter that will keep vaginal tissues healthy. It cranks up your immune system, stimulates growth of healthy vaginal tissues, strengthens cell membranes, and protects the vagina from further infection, says Pamela Jeanne, N.D., a naturopathic doctor and owner of Mount Hood Holistic Health in Gresham, Oregon. But it does have some drawbacks, she notes. If you take too much, it could affect your liver, and if pregnant women take high doses for long periods of time, there's a chance that their babies may have birth defects.

As an alternative, you can take beta-carotene. It helps to produce more vitamin A in your body, but unlike vitamin A, beta-carotene can be taken in large doses without the worry of side effects.

If you have a vaginitis infection, you can take 5,000 to 10,000 international units (IU) of vitamin A daily if you're not pregnant, not trying to conceive, and are using a reliable method of birth control, Dr. Jeanne advises. Alternatively, you can take 100,000 IU of beta-carotene daily, she says. But you need to talk to your doctor if you're taking this much beta-carotene.

Get C and E on your side. Vitamin C kicks your immune system into high gear, strengthening your body's ability to fight off the infection. Vitamin C helps reduce the inflammation and strengthens capillary walls and mucous membranes lining your vagina so they can ward off infection, says Dr. Jeanne. "Make sure the vitamin C you take contains bioflavonoids or rose hips," she says. "Bioflavonoids prevent the infected vaginal cells from releasing immune system chemicals called histamines, which cause the inflammation."

Take 2,000 milligrams of vitamin C daily to maintain a healthy vagina, Dr. Jeanne suggests. If you suffer from chronic vaginal infections, take 3,000 to 4,000 milligrams a day over a 2-week period until symptoms improve.

Vitamin E should be the number one nutrient for women during and after menopause, says Dr. Jeanne. Estrogen levels drop and remain low once menopause is under way, leading to the irritation, inflammation, and other vaginal problems related to low estrogen. Dr. Jeanne believes that vitamin E can lower this risk by strengthening the cell membranes lining your vagina. The stronger the membranes, the less likely it is that bacteria will invade them and wreak havoc.

With your doctor's consent, you can take 400 to 800 IU of vitamin E daily, says Dr. Jeanne. Sometimes, higher dosages are recommended, depending on your condition.

Have some zinc. The mineral zinc is another powerful healer and protector against vaginal infection. It will support your immune system so you can battle the infection. It's vital for the production of collagen, the connective tissue that helps wounds heal, and it can create new skin.

During an infection, take 30 to 60 milligrams of zinc daily in divided doses, says Dr. Jeanne. Since zinc can cause stomach upset, you might want to take a partial dose with each of your meals. You shouldn't take zinc if you have certain health conditions, however, so talk to your doctor before starting these dosages.

Strike a balance with acidophilus. When vaginitis is caused by a yeast overgrowth, the best supplement to take is *Lactobacillus acidophilus*, says Liz Collins, N.D., a naturopathic doctor and co-owner of the Natural Childbirth and Family Clinic in Portland, Oregon. It's the predominant type of bacteria that keeps the vagina healthy and helps keep other vaginal bacteria in balance. Without enough acidophilus, yeast organisms can grow uncontrollably.

Naturopathic doctors believe that acidophilus keeps the yeast population under control by producing lactic acid and natural antibiotic substances. "There is almost always yeast inside the vagina, and that's okay," says Dr. Collins. "The problem starts when your vaginal immune system is weak, and you don't have enough acidophilus in there to maintain a balance in the vaginal flora."

To restore that balance, take three capsules of acidophilus or eat 8 ounces of acidophilus yogurt daily, says naturopathic doctor Tori Hudson, N.D., professor at the National College of Naturopathic Medicine in Portland, Oregon, and author of *Women's Encyclopedia of Natural Medicine*. Continue to take the supplements throughout the infection and for a couple of days afterward, Dr. Hudson says. She recommends taking one capsule a half-hour before each meal with a large glass of water.

To make sure you get the live cultures, which are what you need, buy refrigerated capsules and read the label to make sure that you're getting one to two billion live organisms daily.

Wipe out yeast and bacteria with herbs. To clear up bacterial infections and control yeast, consider garlic or echinacea. Whether you take them together or separately, naturopaths believe that these herbs can muster up a tough defense against bacterial offenders. They also help to restore the natural flora to the vagina, reinforcing the efforts of good bacteria.

Garlic strengthens the immune system so that your body can fight off the infection on its own, plus it has both antifungal and antibacterial properties, says Dr. Hudson. Echinacea also deserves high praise. This powerful immune system stimulant has antiviral powers as well.

During an acute infection, take one or two capsules of garlic daily for 3 to 14 days, or until the infection clears up, says Dr. Hudson. Take two capsules daily for 4 weeks or longer if your infection is chronic. Products that contain at least 4,000 micrograms of allicin may be the most effective, she says.

Take 300 milligrams of echinacea three times a day for at least 1 week, says Dr. Jeanne. When symptoms subside, drop the dosage to 300 milligrams twice a day. Dr. Jeanne says that this dose can be taken for 4 to 6 weeks, but after that it's best to stop for a while.

Try licorice for vaginal dryness. During and after menopause, women produce less estrogen, which is one of the basics needed to prevent vaginal problems. "Estrogen feeds the vaginal tissue and promotes circulation and natural lubrication, which protects the vagina from bacteria," says Dr. Collins.

Herbs can replenish some of the lost estrogen and give you the moisture and protection you need. Naturopathic doctors recommend herbs like licorice, dong quai, and black cohosh. But none of these should be taken by women who are pregnant.

Licorice contains natural estrogen-like compounds and seems to help adjust estrogen in both directions, reducing levels that are too high and increasing them when they're too low.

To relieve vaginal dryness, take 200 to 300 milligrams of licorice two or three times a day for 1 to 2 months, says Dr. Jeanne. For the best effects, she recommends taking black cohosh and dong quai along with the licorice. It's not advisable to take excessive doses, however. High daily doses of herbal licorice for more than 4 to 6 weeks may cause your body to react by retaining too much sodium and water. Doctors warn that high doses of licorice may also lead to high blood pressure or impaired heart or kidney function.

Discover cohosh. Black cohosh also contains estrogen, and studies show that this herb relieves vaginal dryness, hot flashes, and depression. You can combine black cohosh with dong quai to get better results if taking the herbs individually doesn't eliminate symptoms. Dr. Collins suggests taking 250 to 300 milligrams of black cohosh three times a day. If you combine it with dong quai, take up to 4,000 milligrams of each per day for up to 6 months. Some women start with 4,000 milligrams per day and then, once their symptoms are under control, decrease the dose slowly to find the minimum dose that maintains control, says Dr. Collins.

Try a woman's tonic. Herbalists say the Chinese herb dong quai relieves vaginal dryness associated with menopause and menstrual problems. Sometimes promoted as the "female ginseng," this herb is a general tonic for the female reproductive system.

Take 300 milligrams of dong quai two or three times a day along with licorice for 1 to 2 months, says Dr. Jeanne. Be patient: It may take several months before the herb begins to relieve symptoms. You shouldn't take it while you're menstruating, however, since it can increase blood loss. It also contains substances that can cause a rash or severe sunburn if you're exposed to sunlight.

Varicose Veins

Varicose veins can make your legs swell or make them feel heavy and tired. They can also aggravate muscle cramps.

When you have varicose veins, it means that the blood returning to your heart is extremely sluggish. Within the veins, valvelike mechanisms that help maintain upward blood flow aren't doing their job any more. It may get to the point where blood is simply pooling in the veins rather than moving along as it should.

Blood vessel damage can set the stage for thrombosis, or clotting, so be sure to see your doctor for a proper diagnosis. If your veins present a real danger to your health, your doctor may recommend sclerotherapy, a procedure that shuts them off, says Decker Weiss, N.M.D., a naturopathic doctor with the Arizona Heart Institute in Phoenix. While that may seem drastic, Dr. Weiss points out that sclerotherapy could relieve discomfort. "The veins aren't helping you in any way," he says. "They are just creating pain."

Naturopathic doctors also recommend nutrients that help to strengthen blood vessel walls or reduce the likelihood of blood clots that could block the veins. Just be sure to talk to your own doctor before you start taking supplements for this condition.

Take fiber for vein strain. Straining to have a bowel movement puts a lot of pressure on the veins of your lower body, and over time, it can promote the development of varicose veins in your legs, Dr. Weiss says.

To prevent constipation, eat foods that contain a mixture of fiber, such as beans, fruits, vegetables, and whole grains. If you also need to take a fiber supplement, find one that contains both soluble and insoluble fibers, Dr. Weiss advises. Also make sure you drink at least eight glasses of water and other fluids every day.

Break up bumps with bromelain. Bromelain, an enzyme that's extracted from green pineapple, can help prevent the development of the hard and lumpy skin found around varicose veins, says Joseph E. Pizzorno Jr., N.D., president of Bastyr University in Bothell, Washington. It can also help people who have a tendency to develop phlebitis, or blood clots in leg veins.

Try taking 500 to 750 milligrams of bromelain on an empty stomach two or three times a day, Dr. Pizzorno recommends. If you take it with meals, it simply works as a digestive enzyme and is used up in your intestines rather than passed along to your bloodstream.

Keep veins strong with bioflavonoids. Even if you seem destined to get varicose veins, the powerful antioxidant and anti-inflammatory properties of bioflavonoids might help make the walls of your veins stronger, says Stephen T. Sinatra, M.D., a cardiologist and director of medical education for Manchester Memorial Hospital in Connecticut.

If you have varicose veins, you should take about 200 to 300 milligrams of grape seed extract or pycnogenol a day with meals for at least 6 months, says Dr. Sinatra. If your discomfort improves, you can continue taking the supplement indefinitely.

Get your vitamins. Vitamin C is needed to help your body manufacture two important connective tissues, collagen and elastin. "Both of these tissues help to keep vein walls strong and flexible," says Dr. Pizzorno. Vitamin C may be especially important if you bruise easily or have broken capillaries, which may show up on your skin as tiny spider veins, he says. He recommends 500 to 3,000 milligrams of vitamin C daily.

Some doctors also recommend a combination of B vitamins, especially to people who have a history of blood clots. It's particularly important to make sure that you're getting sufficient amounts of folic acid, B_{12}, and B_6, Dr. Weiss says.

"I recommend B vitamins to all my patients with heart or circulatory problems as part of a high-potency multivitamin," says Dr. Weiss. If people have absorption problems, he will suggest B_{12} injections. Otherwise, you can take B-vitamin supplements in pill or capsule form.

Bring on the Es. Vitamin E can also help, Dr. Pizzorno says. "Vitamin E helps keep platelets, blood components involved in clotting, from sticking together and from adhering to the sides of blood vessel walls," he says.

Taking 200 to 600 international units of vitamin E a day should be sufficient, Dr. Pizzorno says. If you've had bleeding problems, however, or are taking prescription anticoagulants to help prevent clotting, get your doctor's okay before you take vitamin E.

Get your gotu kola. The herb gotu kola is particularly good for varicose veins and also has a reputation as an anti-aging herb, says Roberta Bourgon, N.D., a naturopathic doctor at the Wellness Center in Billings, Montana. This herb seems to be able to strengthen the sheath of tissue that wraps around veins, reduce formation of clogging scar tissue, and improve blood flow through affected limbs.

"It's really more of a preventive measure than a cure," says Dr. Bourgon. "If you know you're prone to varicose veins, this can help you slow down or perhaps prevent the problem."

Even if it doesn't help the varicosity itself, gotu kola often improves the symptoms of varicose veins, including pain, numbness, and leg cramps, Dr. Bourgon says. Try taking 60 to 120 milligrams a day in capsules.

Vision Loss

More than 10 million Americans have some degree of visual impairment that can't be completely corrected with glasses. The list of sight stealers is long and varied, with Father Time at the head of the list. As the years pass, the lens inside the eyes can gradually thicken and become opaque with cataracts, leading to cloudy spots, blurriness, blinding halos around lights, and poor night vision.

Time can also take a toll on the macula—the part of the eye responsible for straight-ahead vision. In fact, a lifetime of sun exposure and other factors that break down the blood vessels and tissues that nourish the macula is responsible for most vision loss that occurs past age 60. This wear-and-tear process—called macular degeneration—gradually shrivels the macula and affects the straight-ahead vision needed to see fine detail. People with macular degeneration often find that words look broken and bunched up. Blank holes appear on street signs and in the fine print on food labels. Straight-lined objects like door frames take on a wavy, warped look.

Other causes of vision loss include tears in the retina and eye diseases such as glaucoma and diabetic retinopathy. In glaucoma, fluid builds up inside the eyes, and the increasing pressure damages the optic (eye) nerves. Diabetic retinopathy is a complication of diabetes that damages the blood vessels in the retina.

Once your ophthalmologist has diagnosed your vision problem and prescribed treatment, here's what you can do to make the most of your remaining vision.

Shed lots of light on the subject. "An ideal reading lamp should have a 60- to 100-watt light bulb coated to reduce glare and enclosed in a reflective interior to intensify the light," says Amalia Miranda, M.D., director of the Low Vision Clinic and clinical instructor of ophthalmology at the Oklahoma University Health Sciences Center in Oklahoma City. High-intensity halogen lights are super bright but also hot. It's better to use them with a dimmer adjustment, she says.

Bring the world closer. Magnifiers in all shapes, sizes, and strengths can restore your ability to read and enjoy your surroundings, according to Eleanor Faye, M.D., an ophthalmologic surgeon at the Manhattan Eye, Ear, and Throat Hospital. A handheld magnifier, for example, can help you read books and food labels. And special glasses with built-in telescopic-type lenses can help you read street signs.

Blow up your books. If you can afford the investment, a special closed-circuit TV (read/write machine) can magnify your books on a TV screen up to 60 times their normal size. Large-print publications and books on tape are cheaper alternatives. A simple, yellow plastic sheet over a book page can make words pop up and give contrast, according to Lorraine Marchi, founder and executive director of the National Association for Visually Handicapped (NAVH) in New York City. Other useful

Bilberry for Night Blindness

With night blindness, your eyes are slow to adjust when you move from a brightly lit room into a dim one and you're easily blinded by the glare of headlights. British pilots during World War II found that bilberry jam—made from a type of northern European blueberry—helped counteract night blindness.

You probably won't find bilberries or bilberry jam in your supermarket, but your health food store should have bilberry capsules. Take 100 to 500 milligrams of bilberry twice a day. "Try it right before you go out at night," says Robert Abel Jr., M.D., clinical professor of ophthalmology at Thomas Jefferson University in Philadelphia and author of *The Eyecare Revolution*. "You should notice an effect within 20 minutes or so." Take it for a month or two and see how it works for you. If you find that it's working, you can continue to take one dose of 100 milligrams before you go out at night.

low-vision aids include large telephone dials and high-contrast watch faces. For more information about these products, write to NAVH, 22 West 21st Street, New York, NY 10010.

Become a fruit-and-vegetable fan. Dr. Faye's advice: Eat fruits, vegetables, and other foods rich in zinc and vitamins C, E, and A and beta-carotene (it converts to A in the body). "Ample evidence shows that these antioxidants may counteract the sun-related oxygen damage to the eye's cells and slow down age-related vision loss," she says.

Consider supplements for the eyes. For good measure, take a commercial eye supplement featuring the antioxidants mentioned above. "My patients report improved well-being after taking these nutrients, and many demonstrated improved vision," says Dr. Faye.

Wear blue blockers and a sombrero. Amber-tinted sunglasses may help block out blue light, a component of sunlight that may contribute to age-related vision loss over prolonged periods, says Dr. Miranda. These sunglasses reduce glare and improve contrast, while offering protection from the harmful ultraviolet (UV) rays of the sun, she says. Top your head with a wide-brimmed hat and you have good protection from sun damage to eyes.

Quit smoking. Researchers from Harvard Medical School found that compared with people who never smoked, people who smoke 20 or more cigarettes per day had about twice the risk of cataracts.

Watch for wavy doorways. One way to keep alert to any vision loss from macular degeneration is to regularly test yourself by looking at straight-line objects such as window frames, says Matthew Farber, M.D., an ophthalmologist in private practice in Fort Wayne, Indiana. Let your doctor know if any lines appear distorted, wavy, faded, missing, or shimmery, as if seen through heat waves on a highway.

Don't delay—remove the haze. If cataracts are interfering with your vision, a surgeon can remove the cloudy lens. Clear vision is then possible with the help of a lens implant or special glasses or contacts. Your eyes will remain sun-sensitive, however. "For people who have had cataract surgery, blue-blocking sunglasses and a wide-brimmed hat are recommended," says Dr. Miranda. The latest implants have a special coating to protect against UV rays.

Look into laser surgery. Ultra-powerful high-beam laser light can seal or dissolve eye tissues and halt certain disease-caused vision loss, according to Dr. Faye. In the case of macular degeneration, a laser can sometimes repair leaking areas of the macula. This allows the retina to heal and can slow down the disease, says Dr. Faye. In some types of glaucoma, lasers can make small openings in the iris to relieve built-up pressure.

Get an annual eye exam after age 35. Early on, glaucoma doesn't have any symptoms, but as optic nerve damage progresses, peripheral vision gets blanked out, making it seem as though you're looking through a tube. Regular exams are especially important if glaucoma runs in your family or if you're nearsighted or have diabetes. It's also important for black people, who are more susceptible to glaucoma.

Make eyedrops a daily habit. If you have glaucoma, you'll need to take eye-pressure-controlling medicine faithfully and correctly, says James McGroarty, M.D., associate clinical professor of ophthalmology at State University of New York Health Sciences Center in Brooklyn. Each time you insert the drops, close your eye for 60 seconds. That way you won't lose any of the medicine.

Jump on your two-wheeler. Studies show that when people with raised eye pressure used a stationary bike for 30 minutes three times weekly for 10 weeks, they reduced their eye pressure. "Elevated eye pressure in glaucoma is similar to high blood pressure in heart disease," says Linn Goldberg, M.D., associate professor of medicine at the Oregon Health Sciences University in Portland. "If you control the pressure, you can in many instances help prevent or control the disease."

Follow-up studies showed that the exercise effects were long-lasting, but that the pressure went back up to former levels once the exercise stopped. Do *not* stop taking anti-glaucoma medications on your own, warns Dr. Goldberg. If you want to try exercise as an alternative, work with your doctor to create a program suitable for you and to monitor the pressure in your eyes, he says.

While the official word isn't out yet, some practitioners already believe that it's wise and safe to take supplements for macular degeneration, particularly if you've already been diagnosed with it. Plus, since vitamins and minerals may also play a role in prevention, starting now could be your best bet to maintain healthy eyes. Be sure to get your doctor's approval, though, before you take supplements to treat this condition.

Warts

Despite the old folk wisdom, you can't catch warts from toads. Actually, it's the person next to you in the locker room or the child on the playground swing set who passes you the virus that causes warts.

The virus enters the skin through a cut or scrape and sets up shop. One to 8 months later, you get a wart. Warts are especially likely to grow on your fingers and hands but can also appear on your elbows, face, and scalp. And you can make them spread through shaving, scratching, or rubbing. Sometimes they go away on their own; sometimes they stick around for years. Even if a doctor destroys a wart by applying salicylic acid or freezes it with liquid nitrogen, the virus can remain in your skin and cause new warts to grow. Here are some natural remedies that may help prevent or treat warts.

Stoke up on A and zinc. These nutrients are important for healing and skin repair, says Allan Magaziner, D.O., a nutritional medicine specialist and head of the Magaziner Medical Center in Cherry Hill, New Jersey. Eat more foods high in them, such as carrots, sweet potatoes, tuna, and dandelion greens for A and cooked oysters, lean beef, whole grains, and nuts for zinc.

You may also get relief with this remedy recommended by Elson Haas, M.D., director of the Preventive Medical Center of Marin in San Rafael, California, and author of *Staying Healthy with Nutrition*. In the morning, crush a vitamin A capsule, mix it with just enough water to make a paste, and apply it directly to the wart. In the afternoon, apply a drop of castor oil; in the evening, apply a drop of lemon juice. This should help dissolve the wart.

Image them gone. Close your eyes, breathe out three times, and imagine yourself at a cool, clear mountain stream, writes Gerald Epstein, M.D., a New York City psychiatrist, in his book *Healing Visualizations*. Picture the part of your body that has the wart. Remove the part, turn it inside out, and wash it thoroughly in the stream. Envision all of the waste products as gray or black strands that are carried away in the swift current. Once the body part is clean, hang it out to dry in the sun. Imagine it healing from the inside, looking like all of the healthy cells around it. When it is dry, turn it right-side out, put it back on, and notice that the wart has vanished. Open

When to See a Doctor

- You have a wart that grows in a place that prevents you from normal functioning, such as a fingertip.
- Your wart is painful, bleeds, or changes shape or color.
- Your wart grows bigger than the eraser on a pencil.

your eyes. Do this exercise three times a day, 2 to 3 minutes at a time, for 21 days.

Hypnotize them. It may sound weird, but it can work. Research has shown that 20 to 50 percent of people who can deeply relax and give themselves hypnotic suggestions can eliminate their warts. "It doesn't matter whether you think you are hypnotizable," says Nicholas Spano, Ph.D., a professor of psychology at Carleton University in Ottowa, Ontario. "What makes the suggestion work is your ability to *vividly imagine* your warts flaking off and growing smaller, and your skin feeling warm and tingling as it heals."

Research results indicate that self-hypnosis is even more effective on warts than treatment with salicylic acid, Dr. Spanos says.

Water Retention

People who retain fluid know how easy it is to swell up like a sponge. "Weight fluctuations of as much as 4 to 5 pounds in a single day are not uncommon in women with fluid retention problems," says Marilynn Pratt, M.D., a physician in private practice in Playa del Rey, California, who specializes in women's health.

Bloating occurs when fluid that normally flows through the body in blood vessels, lymph ducts, and tissues gets trapped in tissues in the tiny channels between cells. A high sodium level attracts more fluid from the blood into the cells, where the fluid gets trapped and the cells become overhydrated. This occurs more readily in women, because their tissues are designed to fluctuate or expand for pregnancy.

Lots of things can cause waterlogged tissues: allergic reactions to foods, heart and kidney problems, and prescription drugs such as hormones. In women, hormonal changes often cause bloating beginning 7 to 10 days prior to menstruation, as higher levels of estrogen and progesterone during that part of the cycle cause the body to retain salt (sodium) and therefore to retain fluid in tissues. "Replacement hormones (especially estrogen alone) can also cause substantial bloating and weight gain," says Dr. Pratt.

Usually, fluid retention is uncomfortable but not health-threatening. People who retain fluid because of heart or kidney problems, however, or who are taking diuretics (water pills) need to be under a doctor's care for their problems, says Dr. Pratt.

Nutritional changes like the following may help for normal bloating, say doctors.

Make the salt connection. An evening's overload on movie popcorn or ballpark franks can leave us puffy-eyed and headachy, with stiff, swollen hands and feet the next morning. "That's because our kidneys retain fluid in our bodies so that the excess salt can be diluted," explains David McCarron, M.D., professor of medicine and head of the Division of Nephrology, Hypertension, and Clinical Pharmacology at Oregon Health Sciences University in Portland. Contrary to what you might think, drinking more water will not worsen fluid retention and may even help.

And some researchers believe that too little salt in the diet can also cause fluid retention, Dr. McCarron says. "It may trigger the kidneys to secrete more of a hormone that conserves salt, in part by reducing urinary output," Dr. McCarron says. He recommends keeping salt intake at 2,400 milligrams (a little more than 1 teaspoon) a day, an amount thought to maintain optimum blood pressure.

For most people, this still means cutting back by about 1,000 milligrams (about a half-teaspoon) a day. Since most of our salt comes from processed foods, not from the shaker, the best way to cut back is to look for sodium-free or low-sodium versions of cheeses, nuts, crackers, lunchmeats, canned soups, and vegetables.

Women who are dieting may be eating a lot of celery, which has a higher level of sodium than any other vegetable, Dr. Pratt says. Munch on carrot sticks instead.

Mix and match your minerals. Getting too little potassium, calcium, or magnesium in your diet can also contribute to fluid retention, Dr. McCarron says. "These

5 Ways to Minimize Water Build-up

Here are food-related remedies experts recommend.

Drink more water. If your fluid retention is caused by excess salt intake, cut back immediately and drink plenty of water, at least eight glasses a day, to help flush out the salt, says Marilynn Pratt, M.D., a physician in private practice in Playa del Rey, California.

Watch out for MSG. Monosodium glutamate contains sodium. It's found in Chinese food and lots of processed foods. Look for MSG or hydrolyzed vegetable protein on labels.

Avoid alcohol. Alcohol acts as a diuretic, making you lose excess water, but can lead to dehydration. And it depletes your body of vitamins and minerals.

Try a natural diuretic. Parsley tea has a mildly diuretic effect. Brew 2 teaspoons of dried leaves per cup of boiling water and steep for 10 minutes. Drink up to three cups a day.

Ferret out food allergies. If you wake up in the morning congested, with puffy eyes and a headache, suspect a food allergy, says Joseph Pizzorno Jr., N.D., a naturopathic physician and president of Bastyr University in Seattle. Wheat is the most common allergy-causing food, but it could be any food. So it's best to get tested, he says.

minerals all play important roles in the fluid balance in your body."

He recommends getting about 3,500 milligrams of potassium a day (the Daily Value), an amount you can obtain by eating at least five servings of fruits and vegetables. (Potassium is lost in cooking water, though, so don't count on boiled potatoes or greens for this mineral.)

For magnesium, aim for the Daily Value of 400 milligrams, Dr. McCarron suggests. Most people fall short of this amount. Nuts, legumes, and whole grains supply the most magnesium; other good food sources are green vegetables and bananas.

And for calcium, strive for 1,000 to 1,500 milligrams a day. One quart of skim milk contains about 1,400 milligrams of calcium.

If you have heart, kidney, or liver problems or diabetes or if you're taking a diuretic to relieve fluid retention or high blood pressure, supplement these minerals only under medical supervision to make sure you don't develop dangerously high blood levels, says Dr. McCarron. People who are taking nonsteroidal anti-inflammatory drugs, potassium-sparing diuretics, ACE inhibitors, or heart medications such as heparin should also check with their doctors before supplementing potassium.

Aid hormone-related bloating with B₆. "Vitamin B_6 plays a role in the body's use of several hormones associated with fluid retention, including estrogen and progesterone," says Dr. Pratt. "By helping the body to metabolize these hormones, B_6 may help the liver metabolize excess amounts, which may be present during the premenstrual period."

Dr. Pratt recommends taking 200 milligrams a day (50 milligrams four times a day) for the 5 days before your period begins. Take a B_6 supplement along with a supplement containing the rest of the B-complex vitamins. "These nutrients interact, so they work better when adequate amounts of all are available," Dr. Pratt says.

Vitamin B_6 can be toxic and can cause serious nerve damage in excessive amounts. For these reasons, it's best not to take more than 100 milligrams a day without checking with your doctor. You may, however, safely take up to 200 milligrams daily for 5 days to relieve premenstrual bloating, Dr. Pratt says. If your hands or feet start to feel numb or clumsy, stop taking B_6 and tell your doctor.

Weight Gain

Too bad there's no such thing as a miracle weight-loss pill. If there were, we'd all be showing off our new-found physiques. Ninety-seven million American adults are overweight or obese, and carrying around these extra pounds puts us at risk for diabetes, heart disease, and cancers of the breast, ovaries, uterus, prostate, and colon. The added weight also affects our emotional health.

To avoid these health problems, you must burn more calories than you consume. You can do that by eating healthfully and exercising regularly. That means eating lots of fruits, vegetables, legumes, and whole grains so that your diet derives 30 percent or less of its calories from fat.

You should also get 30 minutes or more of moderate-intensity aerobic exercise such as walking, jogging, or cycling 5 to 7 days a week. Strength training or resistance training helps, too. Working with any kinds of weights increases lean muscle mass, which burns more calories than fat does and speeds up your metabolism.

Once you adopt these strategies, you may find that supplements can also work in your favor. Some can help suppress your appetite, alternative medicine experts say. And some can help increase the rate at which you burn calories.

Fill up with fiber. Just as fiber-rich fruits and vegetables can help you achieve that slender waistline, so can fiber supplements. "Once you take a fiber supplement, it expands in your stomach dramatically, filling you up," says Jennifer Brett, N.D., a naturopathic doctor at the Wilton Naturopathic Center in Stratford, Connecticut. The best fiber supplements are glucomannan and psyllium because they are rich in soluble fiber, says Dr. Brett.

What's more, these supplements have been shown to reduce the number of calories that your body absorbs from food each day, says Liz Collins, N.D., a naturopathic doctor and co-owner of the Natural Childbirth and Family Clinic in Portland, Oregon.

Several studies have shown that fiber supplements can reduce the number of calories absorbed each day by 30 to 180. That adds up to approximately 3 to 18 fewer pounds a year.

Dr. Brett recommends one glucomannan pill 20 minutes before each meal or two or three capsules of psyllium before meals. Drink at least 8 ounces of water with each dose to prevent constipation.

Get lean with chromium. Chromium picolinate can build muscle mass and reduce fat in people who exercise. The more muscle you gain, the more calories you'll burn each day.

Chromium also helps your body turn carbohydrates and fats into energy. Moreover, it improves the effectiveness of insulin, the hormone that allows cells to pick up blood sugar that your body needs for fuel from the bloodstream. As a result, blood sugar levels are kept under control. Your energy soars, you crave fewer sweets, and your body's sensitivity to insulin increases, which is key for successful weight loss, says Dr. Brett. She suggests taking 200 to 400 micrograms of chromium picolinate daily, but doses this high must be taken under medical supervision.

Try an herbal fat burner. Kelp is one herb that may actually help whittle away extra pounds when combined with a low-fat diet and daily aerobic exercise, says Ellen Evert Hopman, a professional member of the American Herbalists Guild, a lay homeopath in Amherst, Massachusetts, and author of *Tree Medicine, Tree Magic.*

Kelp is a type of seaweed that's rich in antioxidant vitamins and iodine. It is believed to stimulate a hormone produced by the thyroid gland that's responsible for boosting metabolism, so you'll burn more calories by the hour, says Hopman. You can also get other kinds of seaweed in your diet by adding them to soups and salads, she says.

If you take kelp, just follow the instructions on the bottle. While it's completely safe for most people, you should check with your doctor before taking it if you have a thyroid disorder, high blood pressure, or heart problems, says Hopman.

Index

Underscored page references indicate boxed text.